广东省本科高校高等教育教学改革项目（粤教高函〔2020〕1 号）

广东省本科高校课程思政示范课程（202122011）

广东省线下一流本科课程（202013059）

暨南大学本科教材资助项目

MPR 出版物链码使用说明

本书中凡文字下方带有链码图标"———"的地方，均可通过"泛媒关联"App 的扫码功能或"泛媒阅读"App 的"扫一扫"功能，获得对应的多媒体内容。

您可以通过扫描下方的二维码下载"泛媒关联"App、"泛媒阅读"App。

"泛媒关联" App 链码扫描操作步骤：

1. 打开"泛媒关联"App；

2. 将扫码框对准书中的链码扫描，即可播放多媒体内容。

"泛媒阅读" App 链码扫描操作步骤：

1. 打开"泛媒阅读"App；

2. 打开"扫一扫"功能；

3. 扫描书中的链码，即可播放多媒体内容。

扫码体验：

腹壁连续缝合术

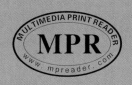

Pathophysiology
Experiments Guidance and
Case Analysis

病理生理学
实验指导及病例分析

主　编：朱丽红

主　审：陆大祥

编　写：（按姓氏笔画排列）

　　　　王一阳　王达安　吕秀秀　李红梅

　　　　张珂珂　彭　爽　魏　伟

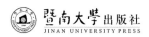

暨南大学出版社
JINAN UNIVERSITY PRESS

中国·广州

图书在版编目（CIP）数据

病理生理学实验指导及病例分析 = Pathophysiology Experiments Guidance and Case Analysis：汉英对照/朱丽红主编. —广州：暨南大学出版社，2022.7
ISBN 978 - 7 - 5668 - 3416 - 4

Ⅰ.①病⋯　Ⅱ.①朱⋯　Ⅲ.①病理生理学—实验—教材—汉、英　Ⅳ.①R363 - 33

中国版本图书馆 CIP 数据核字（2022）第 078422 号

病理生理学实验指导及病例分析
BINGLISHENGLIXUE SHIYAN ZHIDAO JI BINGLI FENXI
主　编：朱丽红

··

出 版 人：张晋升
责任编辑：黄文科　彭琳惠
责任校对：苏　洁
责任印制：周一丹　郑玉婷

出版发行：暨南大学出版社（511443）
电　　话：总编室（8620）37332601
　　　　　营销部（8620）37332680　37332681　37332682　37332683
传　　真：（8620）37332660（办公室）　37332684（营销部）
网　　址：http：//www.jnupress.com
排　　版：广州尚文数码科技有限公司
印　　刷：佛山市浩文彩色印刷有限公司
开　　本：787mm×1092mm　1/16
印　　张：9.25
字　　数：160 千
版　　次：2022 年 7 月第 1 版
印　　次：2022 年 7 月第 1 次
定　　价：39.80 元

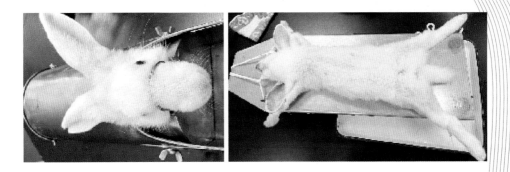

图1　家兔的保定方式

Fig. 1　Fixing of rabbit

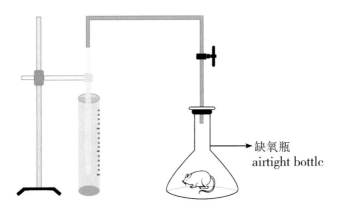

缺氧瓶
airtight bottle

图2　耗氧量测量装置

Fig. 2　Apparatus for measuring oxygen consumption

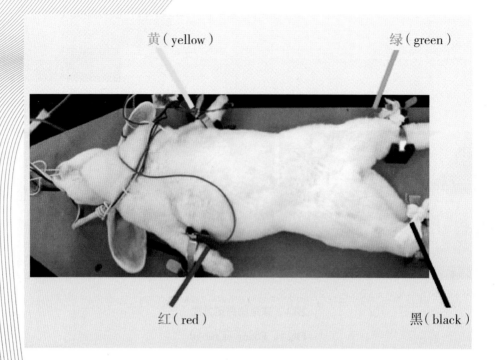

图3　家兔心电导联

Fig. 3　Rabbit ECG lead

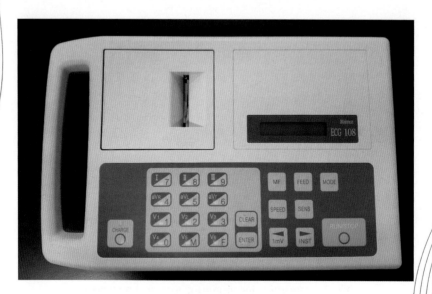

图4　心电图机

Fig. 4　Electrocardiograph（ECG）

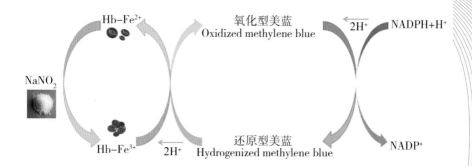

图 5 适量美蓝治疗亚硝酸盐中毒的机理

Fig. 5 Mechanism that treatment of nitrite intoxication by methylene blue at proper dose

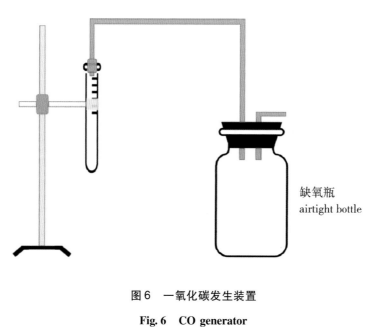

缺氧瓶
airtight bottle

图 6 一氧化碳发生装置

Fig. 6 CO generator

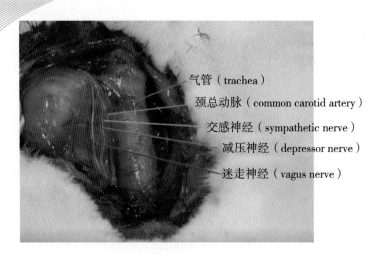

气管（trachea）

颈总动脉（common carotid artery）

交感神经（sympathetic nerve）

减压神经（depressor nerve）

迷走神经（vagus nerve）

图 7　颈部解剖——颈总动脉

Fig. 7　Neck anatomy—Carotid artery

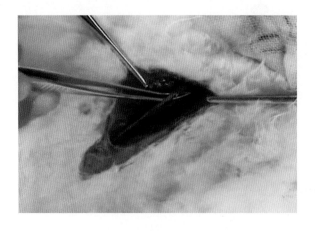

图 8　股三角解剖——股动脉

Fig. 8　Femoral triangle anatomy—femoral artery

目　录

CONTENTS

第一部分 概 论

一、实验课的目的

病理生理学是医学基础理论学科之一，它的任务是研究疾病发生的原因和条件，探讨疾病的发病机制及患病全过程机体的机能代谢变化，从而阐明疾病发生和转归的规律，为疾病的防治提供理论依据。

病理生理学是一门理论性较强的学科，学习者必须认真学习本学科的基本理论，复习相关学科的基础知识，做到融会贯通，运用科学思维正确认识疾病中出现的各种变化，不断提高分析问题和解决问题的能力。

病理生理学又是一门实践性较强的学科，为了研究疾病的发病机制和机体的机能代谢变化，必须进行大量的实验研究。但是大部分的实验研究不能直接在人身上进行，这就需要可以复制人类疾病的动物模型，在动物身上观察其病理生理变化并进行治疗，以探讨疗效机制。动物实验的结果往往为临床实践提供重要的借鉴和参考，可以说，病理生理学的大量成果主要来自实验研究，特别是动物实验。

为此，病理生理学的教学安排了适量的动物实验内容，通过具体的操作与观察和典型病例的课堂讨论，印证所授的部分理论，加深学生对相关理论的理解。实验教学又是对学生独立思考和独立工作能力的训练，通过观察分析科学现象、收集整理实验数据和书写实验报告，使学生初步掌握病理生理学实验的基本操作方法；加强对学生科研素质的培养，训练学生的自学能力、动手操作能力和语言书写表达能力，开拓创新思维，树立严谨求实的科学作风。

二、实验课的基本要求

（1）实验课前要认真预习，了解本次实验的目的要求、方法原理和操作步骤，并复习相关的理论内容。

（2）遵守课堂纪律，不迟到不早退，进入实验室必须穿工作服，上课期间不进行与实验课无关的活动。

（3）爱护公物，严格遵守各种仪器设备的操作规程，注意节约实验用品。

（4）注意安全，防止触电、火灾、污染、中毒及被动物咬伤等事故的发生。如发生实验器材损坏或伤害事故，应及时向教师报告，正确处理。

（5）及时准确、真实客观地记录实验结果，不发生错误或遗漏，不随意修改实验数据，自觉培养严谨的科学作风。

（6）课堂讨论时积极发言，要求语言简练，观点明确，依据充分。

（7）实验结束后整理实验器材，清洗并清点实验器械，做好实验室的清洁卫生工作。

（8）认真书写实验报告，按时交给指导教师评阅。

三、实验报告的书写

实验报告的书写是一项重要的基本技能训练，是科研论文写作的基础，要认真对待，独立完成。

实验报告应做到书写格式规范，文字表达准确、通顺，结果描述客观真实，讨论分析理论联系实际，对实验内容进行推理和思考，提出自己的见解，避免盲目抄书，更不能抄袭他人的实验报告。

实验报告应按如下格式书写：

（1）姓名、年级、班次、组别（可写在实验报告本的封面）。

（2）实验项目与实验日期。

（3）实验目的与原理。

（4）实验对象。

（5）材料与方法。

（6）实验结果：说明实验对象在处理因素的作用下所出现的病理生理效应，可用文字详加描述，也可用图表将经整理后的实验数据列出，并加以文字说明，使之清晰明确、一目了然，便于相互比较。

（7）讨论：针对该次实验结果，解释和分析其发病机制和理论依据，若实验出现了非预期结果，应考虑和分析其原因，分析推理要实事求是，有科学依据，符合逻辑。

（8）小结：应与实验目的相呼应，是从实验结果归纳出来的一般性概括和判断，是该次实验所能验证的理论的简明总结，其文字要精练。

第二部分　实验动物基本操作

一、实验动物的标准化及选择

（一）动物用于实验研究的优越性

动物实验具有易于设置对照、严格控制条件、突出实验因素、避免人为因素的干扰等优点。可使用标准化的实验动物进行在人身上无法进行的实验观察与研究。通过复制人类疾病的动物模型，能大批量、大规模地开展研究，克服病例获取困难的限制，加快研究进程。

（二）动物用于实验研究的局限性

实验动物与人在解剖结构、生理机能、物质代谢、对致病原和药物的敏感性和反应性等方面存在着差别。因此，在无充分依据的情况下，动物实验的结论不应轻易、简单地外推到人身上。人的社会性和心理因素对病理生理机制的影响更是实验动物难以代替的。

（三）实验动物的标准化

标准化实验动物是指遗传背景和生物学特征明确、微生物净化程度清楚、按严格操作程序人工繁育的动物群类。标准化实验动物按遗传背景分类可分为近交系动物（也称纯系动物）、系统杂交动物、封闭群杂种动物和普通杂种动物；按微生物净化程度分类可分为无菌动物、已知菌动物、无特定病原体动物、清洁动物和普通带菌动物。

（四）实验动物的选择

实验动物种类繁多，选用不当可能导致实验失败甚至得出错误结论。事实上，许多人类疾病模型的复制都已经有较为合适的实验动物可供选用，可参照有关文献建模。按照符合实验研究的目的和要求，基于易于饲养管理、经济易得等原则，选用实验动物应注意以下几个方面：

（1）选用与人的结构、机能、代谢和疾病特点相近的动物，如狗的消化系统、猪的皮肤结构与人相似；雌性猕猴的生殖生理周期与人近似等。

（2）根据动物某些功能高度发达、反应特别敏感或解剖结构特殊的特点选用，如狗的神经系统发达、猫对呕吐反应敏感、家兔对发热敏感、金地鼠对钩体感染敏感、家兔颈部减压神经易于分离、大鼠无胆囊等。

此外，应注意对实验动物在年龄、性别、体重、健康状态方面的选择，尽量照顾到实验季节、生物节律等对实验结果的影响。

二、实验动物的捕拿、保定、给药和麻醉

（一）实验动物的捕拿和保定

捕拿和保定是动物实验操作技术的基本功，其原则是要保证实验人员的安全，防止实验动物意外损伤，禁止对实验动物采取粗暴动作。捕拿动作应准确、迅速、熟练，争取在实验动物感到不安之前捕拿稳定。保定是指为使动物实验或其他操作顺利进行而采取方法或设备限制动物行动的操作。保定器具要结构合理、规格适宜、便于操作，在不影响实验操作的情况下，最大限度减少对动物身体的强制限制。捕拿和保定方法因实验动物的不同而变化。

1. 家兔

家兔脚爪锐利，需谨防被抓。一般用右手抓住家兔背部皮肤，轻轻提起，再用左手托住其臀部，使其重量主要集中在左手上。切忌只抓住两只耳朵、拖拉四肢或捕拿腰背部，造成家兔受伤。

常用的保定方式主要为盒式、台式，应根据实验需要选取保定方式。若仅做家兔头部的操作，如耳缘静脉麻醉、取血或注射，可用兔盒保定；若要做家兔颈部、腹部等手术，可用兔台保定，使家兔仰卧，抓住其颈背部和臀部皮肤将其翻转，用棉绳套在其四肢腕或踝关节以上进行保定，再用兔头固定器固定其头部或用粗棉线保定其门齿（见图1）。

2. 小鼠

小鼠性情温和，一般不需要戴手套捉拿，但捉拿时切勿粗暴，防止捏伤小鼠或触怒小鼠。捉拿时，先用右手的拇指和食指捏住小鼠尾巴中部，将小鼠置于鼠笼盖或粗糙面上（切勿悬空），略向后拉，再用左手的拇指、食指和中指抓住小白鼠两耳和颈背部皮肤，使其翻转仰卧于左手大鱼际肌上，以无名指及小指夹住鼠尾根部，将其保定于左手中。如果实验时间过长，也可将小鼠麻醉后固定于小鼠固定板上再进行操作。

（二）实验动物的给药途径和方法

1. 小鼠腹腔注射法

左手保定小鼠，将其头部朝下、腹部朝上，右手持注射器从左下腹部（避免损伤肝脏）向头部方向刺入，45°角进针 2 ~ 3 mm。当感到落空感时，则表明针头已进入腹腔，若回抽无血、肠液或尿液，则可注射。

2. 家兔耳缘静脉注射法

首先将家兔置于保定盒内，注射前去除耳缘静脉注射部位的被毛，用手指轻弹兔耳部，使静脉充盈扩张。左手的食指和中指轻压耳根部，拇指和无名指固定耳缘静脉的远心端，把左手的无名指放在其下作垫，待静脉显著充盈后，右手持针，尽量从静脉远心端刺入，顺着血管平行方向推进 1 cm 后，放松对耳根处血管的压迫。移动左手大拇指去固定针头，缓慢注射药液。注射结束后，拔出针头，用干棉球压迫针孔至不出血为止。

（三）实验动物的麻醉

在急、慢性动物实验中，手术前均应将实验动物麻醉，即利用特定药物对其中枢神经系统进行抑制，以减轻或消除实验动物的痛苦，让其保持安静，确保实验顺利进行。实验动物麻醉方法有全身麻醉和局部麻醉两种，前者又可分为吸入性麻醉和注射麻醉，在病理生理学实验中主要使用注射麻醉。

1. 全身麻醉

常见的注射麻醉剂主要有氨基甲酸乙酯（乌拉坦）、戊巴比妥钠、水合氯醛等。注射麻醉一般采用静脉注射和腹腔注射。腹腔注射麻醉一般将麻醉药总量一次性注入。静脉注射麻醉速度快，兴奋期短，可根据实验动物反应随时调整注射的速度和用量，易于准确达到麻醉深度，是常用的麻醉手段之一。

（1）小鼠：腹腔注射戊巴比妥钠 30～90 mg/（kg·BW）。

（2）家兔：静脉注射25%乌拉坦 5 mL/（kg·BW）。

2. 局部麻醉

局部麻醉通常采用1%普鲁卡因溶液，在手术部位做皮内注射或皮下组织浸润注射，主要用于使动物保持清醒，减少痛苦。

3. 麻醉效果的评估

实验动物麻醉效果的评估可以通过肉眼观察或刺激反应来判断。

（1）麻醉完全：注射麻醉药物后，动物躯体自然倒下，呼吸变深变慢，瞳孔缩小为原来的1/4，角膜反射迟钝，四肢肌肉松弛，此为最佳麻醉效果。

（2）麻醉过量：麻醉药物过量时，动物或呼吸、心跳骤停，或全身青紫、呼吸浅而慢。

（3）麻醉剂量不足：注射麻醉后，动物仍然挣扎、尖叫、对疼痛敏感、呼吸较快等，应观察一段时间，确认达不到所需麻醉深度时，可再次追加剂量，一次不宜超过总量的1/5。

三、常见手术器械的使用

动物实验所用的手术器械分为一般手术器械和显微手术器械。本节介绍一般手术器械的正确握持方法及用途。

1. 手术刀

手术刀由刀柄和刀片组成，主要用于切开皮肤、组织或脏器等。根据手术部位与性质的不同，可选用不同大小和形状的手术刀。持刀方法主要有反挑式、握持式、执笔式、执弓式。装载刀片时，用持针器夹持刀片前端背部，使刀片的缺口对准刀柄前部的刀棱，稍用力向后拉动即可装上。使用后，用持针器夹持刀片尾端背部，提取刀片时稍用力向前推即可将刀片卸下。

传递手术刀时，传递者应握住刀柄与刀片衔接处的背部，将刀柄尾端送至术者手里，不可将刀刃对着术者传递，以免造成损伤。

2. 剪刀

剪刀有尖、钝，直、弯，长、短多种类型。

（1）手术剪：用于剪神经、人体表皮组织或软组织。

（2）组织剪：供剪切组织用。多为弯剪，锐利而精细，用来解剖、剪断或分离组织。通常，直剪适用于浅部操作；弯剪适用于深部操作。

（3）线剪：供剪、拆缝合线用。多为直剪，其与组织剪的区别在于组织剪的刀刃锐薄，线剪的刀刃钝厚。因此坚决不能用组织剪代替线剪，以免损坏刀刃。

（4）眼科剪：用于剪细小的软组织或神经、血管。注意切勿用眼科剪剪皮肤、线、纱布等较硬物质，以免损坏刀刃。

正确把持方式：使用剪刀时，拇指和无名指插入柄的两环，中指放在无名指前方柄上，食指轻压轴节处。拇指、中指和无名指控制剪刀的开闭动作，食指用于稳定和控制剪刀方向。

3. 手术镊

常用的手术镊有有齿镊、无齿镊和眼科镊。有齿镊的头部有可以互相咬合的爪形小齿轮，用于夹持较坚硬的组织，使其不易脱落。无齿镊又称解剖镊，头部钝、厚、无齿、内有横纹，可用于夹持神经、血管、肠壁等较脆弱组织。眼科镊仅用来夹持和分离精细组织。

正确持镊姿势：用食指、中指夹持镊柄中部，从而稳而适度地夹住组织。

4. 止血钳

（1）直头止血钳：用于浅部组织的分离、夹住出血的血管。有齿止血钳用于强韧组织的止血、提起皮肤等，不能用于皮下止血。

（2）弯头止血钳：多用于手术深部止血，不宜用于神经等脆弱组织，以免造成不必要的损伤。

（3）蚊式止血钳：常用于精细的手术或细小的出血点，不宜夹持大块或坚硬组织。

持止血钳方式与手术剪相同。开放时，用拇指和食指夹持住止血钳一个环口，中指和无名指夹持住另一环口，将拇指和无名指稍微用力对顶一下，即可放开止血钳。

5. 持针器

持针器专用于夹持缝针进行缝合，其外形和止血钳类似，但持针器的头部齿槽较短且通常内有槽，虽然也有内无槽的。

6. 缝针与缝线

缝针与缝线用于缝合各种组织。缝针有圆针和三棱针两种，又有弯、直之别。圆针对组织创伤较小，多用于软组织的缝合。三棱针常用于皮肤、坚硬组织的缝合。持针器夹持缝针时，用尖端夹住缝针的中后1/3交界处为宜。

7. 动脉夹

动脉夹用于阻断动脉血流。

四、常用的基本外科操作

1. 备皮

将动物麻醉保定后，确定备皮部位与范围，备皮范围应大于手术切口的长度。常用的备皮方法为剪毛法和拔毛法。

（1）剪毛法。

绷紧手术部位皮肤，右手持弯手术剪平贴于动物皮肤，逆着动物毛的朝向剪毛。剪毛时勿用手提起被毛，以防剪破皮肤。将剪下的毛立即放入盛水的容器中浸湿，以免其乱飞。

（2）拔毛法。

兔耳缘静脉注射时，用拇指轻轻拔去所需实验部位的被毛。

2. 皮肤切开方法

（1）剪口法。

术者左手持止血钳提起预剪口处一侧皮肤，助手持止血钳在对侧提起对应位置皮肤，术者持手术剪在被提起皮肤间上下剪开皮肤至所需手术切口长度。剪开皮肤时，注意避开血管部位。

（2）切口法。

根据实验需求确定手术切口的部位、大小及深浅等。切开组织前，先用左手手指将预定切口处皮肤拉紧，使其紧绷，手术刀垂直刺入皮肤，呈45°角运刀，垂直止刀，用力得当，一次性切开皮肤全层。组织要逐层切开，注意止血，尽可能使切口方向与切口下各层组织的纤维方向一致。组织切开的部位应优先选择无重要血管或无神经纵横交贯的地方，尽量避免切断血管和神经，以免引起严重的后果。

3. 组织分离法

（1）锐性分离。

使用剪、刀等锐性器械直接切割分离，用于皮肤、黏膜、组织的精细解剖和紧密粘连组织的分离。

（2）钝性分离。

使用止血钳、手指等分离肌肉、筋膜间隙的疏松结缔组织。软组织要求逐层分离，保持视野清晰，原则上以钝性分离为主，避开血管。

4. 止血方法

手术过程中要立即止血，防止继续失血，保持手术视野清晰。常用的止血方法有压迫止血法、钳夹止血法和结扎止血法。压迫止血法多适用于毛细血管渗血，止血时用温热的纱布按压出血处。钳夹止血法通常适用于阻止小血管出血。对于较大血管出血，常用结扎止血法，先用止血钳夹住出血处，然后用丝线结扎（注意：打结时一定要打紧，避免打假结）。若出血较多，可用温热纱布吸净血液后，看准出血部位再用止血钳夹住。使用止血钳时，应准确夹住出血的血管壁处，尽可能避免夹住血管周围的组织，切不可夹住大块组织。

5. 基本外科手术

下面以家兔为实验对象，说明各种基本外科手术操作步骤。

（1）气管分离和插管术。

将家兔麻醉、保定、备皮，用手术刀沿颈部正中线在甲状软骨与胸骨之间做一5~7 cm切口，暴露胸骨舌骨肌，用止血钳沿其中线插入左右胸骨舌骨肌，做钝性分离。将左右胸骨舌骨肌向两侧拉开，暴露气管。在喉头以下，用弯头止血钳将气管与背后的结缔组织分离一段，穿粗棉线备用。提起棉线，在甲状软骨下2 cm处的两软骨环之间，用剪刀将气管前段横向剪开（占气管壁1/3~1/2），再向头端做一0.5 cm纵切口，使之呈"倒T"字形。将气管插管由切口向心端插入气管腔内，用备用线结扎，再将结扎线固定于"Y"形气管插管分叉处，以防插管脱出。插入插管后要检查管内有无出血，以保证家兔呼吸道顺畅。

（2）颈总动脉分离和插管术。

颈总动脉插管的目的：测量动脉血压或放血。

将家兔麻醉、保定、备皮，用手术刀沿颈部正中线在甲状软骨与胸骨之间做一5~7 cm切口，暴露胸骨舌骨肌，用止血钳沿其中线插入左右胸骨舌骨肌，做钝性分离。将左右胸骨舌骨肌向两侧拉开，暴露气管。颈总动脉位于气管两侧，分离时用止血钳沿胸骨乳突肌前缘分离胸骨舌骨肌与胸骨甲状肌之间的结缔组织（即Y形沟内），在肌缝下找到呈粉红色较大的血管，手触之有搏动感，即为颈总动脉。用浸湿生理盐水的棉球顺着血管走向轻轻拭去血液鞘膜，沿血管走向分离颈总动脉2~3 cm，在其下穿两根生理盐水浸湿的丝线备用。手术过程中要使手术部位保持湿润，擦去血液。

结扎颈总动脉远心端，用动脉夹夹住动脉近心端，在靠近远心端的结扎处稍下方用眼科剪在动脉剪一与血管呈45°角的V形切口（切口大小约为管径1/3），然后用远心端的细线将导管再次固定。

注意：动脉导管插管前，使导管内充满0.3%肝素钠溶液，并将三通置于45°角的关闭状态。

（3）颈外静脉分离和插管术。

颈外静脉插管的目的：注射、取血、输液及中心静脉压的测量。

颈外静脉位置浅，位于颈部皮下。麻醉家兔后，将其仰卧位固定，正中切一6~8 cm长的皮肤切口，用左手拇指和食指提起一侧皮肤，其余手指从皮肤外侧顶起，将皮肤外翻，可见暗紫色的粗大血管——颈外静脉。用钝头止血钳沿血管走向将静脉周围的结缔组织轻轻分离（分离过程中切忌过分牵拉，更不能使用手术刀、手术剪进行分离，以免造成血管破裂），分离长度约为2.0 cm，穿两根生理盐水浸润的丝线备用。

插管前，先准备好导管，插入端剪一斜面，另一端连接于装有生理盐水的输液装置上，让导管内充满溶液。插管方法与颈总动脉插管方法相似，单纯输液时，送入血管的导管长度一般为2~3 cm即可。如测量中心静脉压时，则需插入5 cm，此时导管口在上腔静脉近右心房入口处。

(4) 股动脉分离和插管术。

股动脉分离与插管的目的：分离股动脉、股静脉，进行股动脉、股静脉插管，以备放血、输血、输液、注射药物使用。股动脉、股静脉和股神经位于后肢内侧股三角区的皮肤和一层筋膜之下。

将家兔麻醉后，使其仰卧位固定，在股三角区剪毛备皮。用手触摸股动脉的搏动，沿动脉走向做一 3~5 cm 长的皮肤切口。用止血钳钝性分离皮下组织及筋膜，即可看到股动脉、股静脉和股神经。股静脉位于内侧，股神经位于外侧，而股动脉的位置在中间稍偏后，恰被股神经和股静脉所遮盖。

先用蚊式钳小心分离股神经，然后再钝性分离股动脉与股静脉之间的结缔组织（注意勿损伤血管小分支），将股动脉段分离出长 2~3 cm 的一段，在其下穿两根生理盐水浸润的细线备用。插管方法同颈部血管。

第三部分 综合性实验

实验一 影响缺氧耐受性的因素

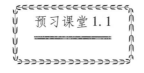

一、实验目的

通过改变机体神经系统机能状态、机体代谢状态及外界环境温度，了解条件因素在缺氧发病机制中的重要性。

二、实验原理

疾病的发生除与病因有直接关系外，各种体内外因素也可影响疾病的发生、发展。机体对缺氧的耐受性除了受缺氧程度和发生速度的影响外，还与其他许多因素如性别、生物节律、机体代谢、神经系统机能状态以及环境温度等有关。这些因素均可作为条件因素影响缺氧作用的后果，有的能增强机体对缺氧的耐受性，有的则加重缺氧的致病作用。本实验通过观察环境温度、机体代谢和神经系统机能状态对乏氧性缺氧小鼠缺氧耐受性的影响，一方面加深对条件因素在疾病发生中作用的理解，另一方面从中选择防治缺氧的最适条件，增强机体对缺氧的耐受能力。

三、实验材料

1. 实验动物

小鼠。

2. 材料

（1）仪器及器材：缺氧瓶；弹簧夹；耗氧量测量装置（图 2）；粗天平；1 mL 注射器；镊子；恒温水浴锅；搪瓷量杯。

（2）试剂：钠石灰；碎冰块；生理盐水；0.7% 戊巴比妥钠；4 mg/100 mL 异丙肾上腺素 +1 g/100 mL 尼可刹米混合溶液。

四、实验步骤

（一）环境温度变化对缺氧耐受性的影响

（1）取缺氧瓶 3 个，各放入钠石灰（大约 5 g）1 包。

（2）取体重相近的小鼠 3 只，称重后分别放入 3 个缺氧瓶中，编号 A、B、C 后作如下处理：

①A 瓶浸入盛有冰块及水的搪瓷量杯中；

②B 瓶浸入 40 ℃ ~42 ℃的水浴锅中；

③C 瓶置室温下。

塞紧瓶塞，弹簧夹夹闭胶管后开始计时。

（3）观察小鼠在瓶中的活动情况，直至小鼠死亡，记录小鼠存活时间并立即从冰水和恒温水浴锅中取出缺氧瓶，置室温中平衡 15 分钟。用耗氧量测量装置测定瓶内总耗氧量。

（4）根据小鼠体重（W）、存活时间（t）、总耗氧量（A），计算小鼠耗氧率（R）。

$$R \ (\text{mL/g} \cdot \text{min}) = \frac{A \ (\text{mL})}{W \ (\text{g}) \cdot t \ (\text{min})}$$

（二）机体状况不同对缺氧耐受性的影响

（1）取缺氧瓶 3 个，各放入钠石灰 1 包。

（2）取体重相近的小鼠 3 只，称重，编号 A_1、B_1、C_1 后分别作如下处理：

①小鼠 A_1：腹腔注射浓度为 4 mg/100 mL 异丙肾上腺素 ＋1 g/100 mL 尼可刹米混合溶液 0.1 mL/10 g 体重。

②小鼠 B_1：腹腔注射 0.7% 戊巴比妥钠 0.1 mL/10 g 体重。

③小鼠 C_1：腹腔注射生理盐水 0.1 mL/10 g 体重。

（3）5 分钟后，将 3 只小鼠分别放入盛有钠石灰的缺氧瓶中，密闭缺氧瓶后开始计时。

（4）观察小鼠在瓶中的活动情况，直至小鼠死亡，记录小鼠存活时间。

（5）按实验步骤（一）中第（4）项的公式计算小鼠耗氧率（R）。

五、注意事项

（1）缺氧瓶一定要保证密闭（可在瓶与瓶塞、瓶塞与玻璃管的缝隙间用吸管注入少量清水，以加强缺氧瓶的密闭效果）。

（2）小鼠腹腔注射应稍靠近左下腹，勿损伤肝脏，也应避免将药液注入肠腔或膀胱。

（3）测量耗氧量时，记录耗氧量测量装置外管（量筒）液面下降的高度。

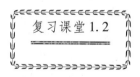

复习课堂 1.2

六、思考题

（1）本实验中引起小鼠死亡的原因是什么？

（2）影响机体缺氧耐受性的因素有哪些？它们是如何起作用的？

附录1：测量耗氧量

一、原理

小鼠在密闭的缺氧瓶内不断消耗氧气，产生的 CO_2 又被钠石灰所吸收，反应如下：

$$NaOH \cdot CaO + H_2O + CO_2 \longrightarrow NaHCO_3 + Ca(OH)_2$$

瓶内氧分压逐渐降低而产生负压，当缺氧瓶与耗氧量测量装置相连时，移液管内液面因缺氧瓶内的负压而上升，量筒液面则下降，下降的体积即为总耗氧量。

二、方法与步骤

（1）向量筒内充水至最大刻度，用乳胶管将耗氧量测量装置与缺氧瓶相连，如图2所示。

（2）打开乳胶管上的弹簧夹，待移液管内液面上升稳定后，从量筒上读出液面下降的毫升数即为小鼠的总耗氧量。

附录2：记录表格

分组		处理	体重 W（g）	存活时间 t（min）	总耗氧量 A（mL）	耗氧率 R（mL/g·min）
一	A	冰水				
	B	40 ℃～42 ℃				
	C	室温				
二	A_1	异丙肾上腺素＋ 尼可刹米混合溶液				
	B_1	戊巴比妥钠				
	C_1	生理盐水				

实验二　高钾血症

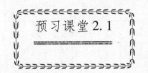

一、实验目的

（1）建立高钾血症动物模型。

（2）观察高血钾症对家兔心脏的毒性作用。

（3）掌握患高血钾症时心电图改变的特征。

（4）了解治疗高钾血症的基本原则。

二、实验原理

通过给家兔静脉注射氯化钾溶液，人为造成家兔血清钾浓度急剧升高（血清钾浓度 >5.5 mmol/L）。同时，通过观察家兔注射氯化钾溶液前后心电图的变化，了解高钾血症对心脏的毒性作用，了解对高钾血症的治疗原则。

三、实验材料

1. 实验动物

家兔。

2. 材料

（1）仪器及器材：心电图机；小儿头皮针；注射器；兔台。

（2）试剂：3%戊巴比妥钠；肝素钠注射液；1%氯化钾；0.1%肝素生理盐水等。

四、实验步骤

（1）家兔称重后，用3%戊巴比妥钠（1 mL/kg）经耳缘静脉注射进行全身麻醉，然后将其仰卧固定于兔台上。

（2）在心电图机导联线原有的圆柱形电极杆外面套上注射针头，将其改装为心电图针形电极，分别插入四肢踝部皮下。导联线按右前肢（红）、左前肢（黄）、右后肢（黑）、左后肢（绿）的顺序连接，见图3。

（3）经耳缘静脉注射 1 mL 肝素钠注射液（12 500 U/2 mL）对家兔进行全身肝素化。

（4）将小儿头皮针与注射器相连，排气后穿刺耳缘静脉，用胶布将头皮针固定在耳廓上，调节输液速度 <10 滴/分，以保持输液管道通畅。

（5）打开心电图机，选择 Ⅱ 导联或 avF 导联记录一段正常心电图，纸长以实验小组内每人能分到 3~4 个完整心电波形为度。

（6）根据家兔的状况，从低剂量开始调节输液速度为 50~60 滴/分，持续静脉滴注 1% 氯化钾溶液，每隔 3 分钟记录一次心电图，直至典型的高钾血症心电图出现。

（7）继续维持滴注 1% 氯化钾溶液，观察心电图波形变化至出现心室颤动或心跳停止为止。

（8）开胸观察心室颤动或心跳停止的状态。

五、注意事项

（1）注射戊巴比妥钠的速度要慢，若过快会导致动物呼吸抑制而死亡。

（2）动物对注入氯化钾的耐受性有个体差异，有的动物需注入较多的氯化钾才出现心电图改变。

（3）注射氯化钾时速度不能太快，尤其是在注射高浓度氯化钾时，速度太快，极易造成动物心脏抑制而死亡，从而无法观察到典型心电图。

（4）耳缘静脉注射应从远心端开始穿刺，如经多次穿刺耳缘静脉已无法注射时，可由股静脉插管注射。

（5）留置的小儿头皮针及注射器内壁应肝素化，以防止出现凝血。

（6）每次使用针形电极时，要用酒精或生理盐水擦净，并及时清除电极和电线周围的血和水迹，以保持良好的导电状态。

（7）描记心电图时应注意避免周围电磁干扰，防止动物挣扎，若动物挣扎过于频繁，可经耳缘静脉追加少量麻醉药，待其安定后才开始记录，以防止损坏心电图机。

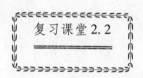

复习课堂2.2

六、思考题

（1）高钾血症对心脏有何影响？

（2）注射氯化钾后，有哪些异常心电图改变？它们是怎样发生的？

（3）最后出现心室颤动时，开胸看到心脏停搏是在舒张期还是在收缩期？为什么？

附录3：心电图机使用的操作步骤

（1）确认心电图机（见图4）地线已接好，按下"POWER"键，打开心电图机电源开关。

（2）将面板上触摸按钮"PROG"置于"MANUAL STD"，将走纸速度"5 25 50"设置为"25"（25 mm/s），将电压"5 10 20"设置为"10"（0.1 mV/格）。

（3）打开"HF"键（高频滤波）和"DF"键（漂移滤波），关闭"MF"键（肌电滤波）。

（4）将"PROG"置于"MANUAL STD"，选择"Ⅱ"导联或"avF"导联。

（5）选择"RUN/STOP"键，按下即可开始描记心电图。停止描记时，再次按下"RUN/STOP"键即可。

实验三 发 热

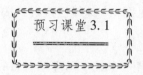

预习课堂 3.1

一、实验目的

（1）建立内毒素及内生致热原发热模型。

（2）观察内毒素及内生致热原发热时体温变化的规律。

（3）观察内毒素及内生致热原的耐热性。

二、实验原理

内毒素是革兰氏阴性细菌细胞壁的化学结构，其活性成分为脂多糖。其耐热性比较强，需置于 160 ℃下 2 小时干热才能灭活。内毒素作为发热激活物，进入机体激活产致热原细胞，产生和释放内生致热原，从而改变体温调定点引起发热。家兔的内毒素发热可呈典型的双相性变化（0.5 μg/kg），第一峰在注入内毒素 1 小时左右，第二峰在 3 小时左右，两峰之间（约 2 小时）有体温下降期。内毒素发热的热程在 6 小时左右。

内生致热原是一种小分子蛋白质，不耐热，90 ℃下 30 分钟即能灭活。内生致热原致热的潜伏期和热程较内毒素短；一般剂量只引起单相热，特大剂量（40 mL/kg）可致双相热。

三、实验材料

1. 实验动物

家兔，体重 2.0～3.0 kg，雌雄不拘。

2. 材料

（1）仪器及器材：婴儿称；测温仪；发热实验记录纸；恒温水浴装置；

注射器；7 号针头。

（2）试剂：液体石蜡；无热原生理盐水；内毒素生理盐水（0.2 μg/mL）；内生致热原溶液。

四、实验步骤

（1）对经适应后体重相近的 5 只健康家兔称量体重，分别标记为 A、B、C、D、E。

（2）将测温探头插入家兔直肠测量直肠温度，每 10 分钟测量 1 次，共测量 3 次，将 3 次的平均值作为基础体温。

（3）分别经耳缘静脉注射不同试剂，并记录注射时间：

①A 兔注入经 38 ℃水浴 30 分钟的无热原生理盐水 5 mL/kg。

②B 兔注入经 38 ℃水浴 30 分钟的内毒素生理盐水 5 mL/kg。

③C 兔注入先经 90 ℃加热 30 分钟，后经 38 ℃水浴 30 分钟的内毒素生理盐水 5 mL/kg。

④D 兔注入经 38 ℃水浴 30 分钟的内生致热原溶液 5 mL/kg。

⑤E 兔注入先经 90 ℃加热 30 分钟，后经 38 ℃水浴 30 分钟的内生致热原溶液 5 mL/kg。

（4）注射后每 5 分钟测量 1 次体温，1 小时后改为每 10 分钟记录 1 次，观察 30 分钟。

（5）分别计算各家兔的体温反应指数（TRI）和体温反应高度（ΔT），比较各家兔的发热效应（计算方法见附录 4）。

五、注意事项

（1）维持实验室温度于 22 ± 2 ℃。

（2）测温探头插入前应用少许液体石蜡或凡士林润滑，以免损伤肛门和直肠。

（3）测温探头插入直肠的深度约 10 cm，并在探头上做标记，以保证插入深度一致。

（4）由于时间关系，发热实验一般只观察 90 分钟，因此看不到内毒素发热的双相热，也看不到内毒素和内生致热原发热的全过程。

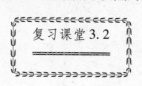

复习课堂 3.2

六、思考题

（1）内毒素发热和内生致热原发热有何规律（潜伏期、热型、热程）？

（2）内毒素与内生致热原的耐热性有何不同？

（3）内生致热原在发热机制中的作用是什么？

附录4：体温反应指数（*TRI*）与
体温反应高度（ΔT）的计算方法

1. 体温反应指数的计算方法

以体温变化值为纵坐标，5 cm = 1.0 ℃；以时间值为横坐标，1.0 cm = 10 min。以注射前3次体温的平均值（四舍五入法，取小数点后一位有效数字）为两坐标的交点，横坐标即为体温基线，上升值为正，下降值为负。在坐标纸上将各时间点体温变化数值描绘成体温变化曲线（发热时为发热曲线）。体温变化曲线与体温基线之间的面积即体温反应指数（发热时即为发热指数），体温反应指数是一种较好反映发热效应强度的指标。

将90分钟内所测各点分别与横坐标做垂直线，可将发热曲线与体温基线之间的面积划分成9个小梯形或三角形。分别计算其面积，9个面积的总和即1.5小时的体温反应指数（cm^2），以 $TRI_{1.5}$ 表示之。

2. 体温反应高度的计算方法

体温反应高度为体温上升的最高值与基线体温之差。体温反应高度是另一种反映发热效应的指标。

附录5：内生致热原的制备

（1）将健康家兔仰卧固定于兔台，在无菌、无内毒素污染条件下操作。

（2）局麻后暴露颈总动脉，经耳缘静脉注入肝素钠溶液 6 250 U（12 500 U/2 mL）。

①用 16 号针头接输液胶管经颈总动脉放血，置于 100 mL 制剂瓶内，再加入肝素钠溶液 2 滴（用 7 号针头）。

②以 2 000 转/分钟离心 20 分钟后吸取上清液（血浆），计量并弃之，补入与血浆等量的生理盐水悬浮沉淀细胞。

③加入 1 μg/mL 精制大肠杆菌内毒素生理盐水溶液（2 mL/100 mL 血液）。

④置于 38 ℃恒温水浴振荡器中孵育 18 小时。

⑤以 2 000 转/分钟离心 20 分钟。

⑥取上清液（含内生致热原）置于 100 mL 制剂瓶内，置于 4 ℃冰箱保存备用。

实验四　缺　氧

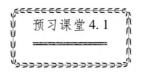

预习课堂 4.1

一、实验目的

（1）建立乏氧性缺氧和血液性缺氧模型。

（2）观察不同类型缺氧对呼吸的影响和血液颜色的变化。

二、实验原理

（一）乏氧性缺氧

引起乏氧性缺氧的原因有吸入气氧分压降低和外呼吸功能障碍等，其共同特征是动脉血氧分压低于正常范围，氧含量、血氧饱和度均降低。本实验将小鼠放入盛有少量钠石灰（$NaOH \cdot CaO$）的密闭缺氧瓶内（见图 2），由于瓶内氧气逐渐被小鼠消耗，而呼出的二氧化碳被钠石灰吸收，因此缺氧瓶内空气的氧分压逐渐降低，而不伴有二氧化碳浓度的增加，此种类型的缺氧为乏氧性缺氧。

（二）血液性缺氧

由于血红蛋白（Hb）数量减少或性质改变，血液携氧能力下降，从而引起组织供氧不足而导致的缺氧为血液性缺氧。

（1）一氧化碳（CO）中毒：按图 2 装置使小鼠吸入 CO，CO 与 Hb 结合后形成碳氧血红蛋白（Hb - CO），从而使 Hb 失去与氧结合的能力而引起缺氧。

（2）亚硝酸钠（$NaNO_2$）中毒：$NaNO_2$ 为强氧化剂，其进入体内使 Hb 分子中的二价铁离子（Fe^{2+}）被氧化为三价铁离子（Fe^{3+}），形成高铁血红蛋白

（MHb），从而使 Hb 失去结合氧的能力。

$$Hb - Fe^{2+} \xrightarrow{NaNO_2} Hb - Fe^{3+}$$

本实验将 $NaNO_2$ 溶液注入小鼠腹腔内，复制亚硝酸钠中毒性缺氧模型，同时取另一只小鼠，用美蓝作为还原剂对抗 $NaNO_2$ 的作用，使被氧化的 Fe^{3+} 还原为 Fe^{2+}，恢复血液携氧能力，一方面反证 $NaNO_2$ 的氧化作用，另一方面探讨 $NaNO_2$ 中毒的解救原理（见图5）。

$$Hb - Fe^{3+} \xrightarrow{美蓝} Hb - Fe^{2+}$$

三、实验材料

1. 实验动物

小鼠。

2. 材料

（1）仪器及器材：缺氧瓶；一氧化碳发生装置（见图6）；2 mL 和 5 mL 移液管；镊子；1 mL 注射器；剪刀。

（2）试剂：钠石灰（$NaOH \cdot CaO$）；甲酸；浓硫酸；5% 亚硝酸钠；1% 美蓝；生理盐水。

四、实验步骤

（一）乏氧性缺氧

（1）取小鼠一只，放入已盛有钠石灰（约5 g）的缺氧瓶中，观察小鼠的一般情况、呼吸频率（次/10 秒）、呼吸深度、皮肤和口唇的颜色，然后塞紧瓶塞，记录时间，以后每3分钟重复观察上述指标一次，直至小鼠死亡。

（2）小鼠尸体留待全部实验完成后，再打开其腹腔，比较血液或肝脏的颜色。

（二）血液性缺氧

1. 一氧化碳中毒性缺氧

（1）如图6设置好一氧化碳发生装置。

（2）将小鼠放入缺氧瓶中，观察记录其呼吸频率和一般表现。

（3）取 3 mL 甲酸放入试管内，再加入 2 mL 浓硫酸，塞紧瓶塞，将已盛有小鼠的缺氧瓶与一氧化碳发生装置相连接。

（4）观察指标与方法同实验步骤（一）中（1）。

2. 亚硝酸钠中毒性缺氧

（1）取体重相近的两只小鼠，观察其正常表现后，分别作如下处理：甲鼠腹腔注射 0.3 mL 5% 亚硝酸钠后，立即再注入 0.3 mL 1% 美蓝溶液；乙鼠腹腔注射 0.3 mL 5% 亚硝酸钠后，立即再注入 0.3 mL 生理盐水。

（2）观察指标与方法同实验步骤（一）中（1）。

（三）比较正常小鼠和上述三只不同缺氧小鼠血液或肝脏的颜色

（1）取正常小鼠 1 只，颈椎脱臼处死，剖开腹腔作正常对照。

（2）分别剖开各缺氧小鼠尸体的腹腔，观察比较各小鼠血液或肝脏的颜色。

五、注意事项

（1）缺氧瓶一定要密封，可用吸管将水加在瓶与塞之间、塞与玻璃管之间的缝隙上，以增加缺氧瓶的密封程度。

（2）小鼠腹腔注射应稍靠近左下腹，勿损伤肝脏，也应避免将药液注入肠腔或膀胱。

（3）一氧化碳产生后应立即与已盛有小鼠的缺氧瓶相连，否则一氧化碳挥发将影响实验效果。切勿将与大气相通的玻璃管封闭，以免产生危险。

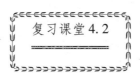

复习课堂 4.2

六、思考题

（1）各类型缺氧的血液颜色变化有何不同，为什么？

（2）各类型缺氧的呼吸变化有何不同，为什么？

（3）各类型缺氧的血气变化有何特点？其发生机制是怎样的？

实验五　失血性休克及其抢救

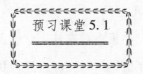

预习课堂 5.1

一、实验目的

（1）建立复制家兔失血性休克模型。

（2）探讨失血性休克的发病机制。

二、实验原理

休克发生的始动环节有：①有效循环血量减少；②心泵功能障碍；③外周血管床容量扩大。临床上有多种原因可引起休克，失血性休克是其中常见的一种。当失血量达到总血量 20% 时，可因循环血量减少出现休克。本实验用人工放血的方法使家兔血压较长时间维持在正常血压的 50%，从而建立家兔失血性休克模型，然后采取不同的救治措施，达到加深理解休克发病机制的目的。

三、实验材料

1. 实验动物

家兔。

2. 材料

（1）仪器及器材：兔台；BioLab – 410 生物机能实验系统；压力换能器；呼吸传感器；手术器械一套；动脉夹；动脉插管；三通；塑料管；5 ~ 10 mL 注射器；50 mL 注射器（放血用）。

（2）试剂：1% 普鲁卡因；3% 戊巴比妥钠；肝素；0.1% 肝素生理盐水；

去甲肾上腺素；山莨菪碱（654 – 2）。

四、实验步骤

（1）取家兔 1 只称重，耳缘静脉注射 1 mL/kg 3% 戊巴比妥钠，麻醉后将其仰卧固定于兔台上。

（2）颈部及一侧下肢内侧备皮，采用 3 ~ 5 mL 1% 普鲁卡因进行局麻。

（3）分离一侧颈总动脉（见图 7），结扎远心端，近心端动脉下穿线打好活结备用。分离气管，在甲状软骨下 0.5 ~ 1 cm 处做"⊥"形切口（可酌情使用局麻）。

（4）分离已备皮侧下肢股动脉（见图 8），结扎远心端，近心端动脉下穿线备用。

（5）行气管插管术，连接呼吸传感器至 BioLab – 410 生物机能实验系统。

（6）耳缘静脉注射肝素 1 mL/只。

（7）行颈总动脉插管（管内充满肝素生理盐水），通过压力换能器连接 BioLab – 410 生物机能实验系统。行股动脉插管（管内充满肝素生理盐水），连接 50 mL 注射器放血用。

（8）记录一段正常血压、呼吸曲线，观察口唇颜色以及测量皮肤温度。

（9）血压平稳 5 分钟后，经股动脉放血至 3/4 基础血压值，停止放血，观察机体代偿性反应和血压变化 10 分钟。

（10）继续经股动脉放血至 40% 基础血压值，维持该血压 30 分钟。

（11）经股动脉插管注射去甲肾上腺素 2 mL（浓度为 75 μg/mL），观察血压的变化。至血压回降至注射前血压值时，行第二次注射，观察血压的变化。至血压回降至注射前血压值时，再行第三次注射。比较三次注射的血压反应。

（12）经股动脉插管注射 654 – 2（10 mg/只），观察血压的变化。

（13）经股动脉回输全部放出的动脉血，观察血压的变化至平稳。

（14）再次经股动脉插管注射 654 – 2（10 mg/只），观察并比较两次注射 654 – 2 血压的变化特点。

实验全程观察并记录血压、呼吸、口唇颜色以及皮肤温度的变化。

五、注意事项

（1）戊巴比妥钠麻醉时需慢推，过快会引起呼吸抑制。

（2）动脉插管使用前一定要充满肝素生理盐水；50 mL 注射器使用前须经肝素生理盐水灌洗，以防止凝血。

（3）手触摸到股动脉搏动后，在该位置行股内侧皮切开，分离股动脉。股动脉、股静脉、股神经三者并行，通常股动脉居中。

（4）插管时应注意：

①插管前先检查外套塑料管尖端是否破损；

②插管进针处要尽可能靠近动脉远心端；

③插管一经进入动脉 2 mm，助手应马上拔出针，同时术者固定好插管，以防脱落；

④继续插入 1 cm 后，用缝线结扎固定。

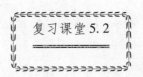

复习课堂 5.2

六、思考题

（1）如何判断休克的发生？有哪些体征可帮助诊断？

（2）在休克发生发展中，三个始动环节是如何起作用的？三者之间有何关联？

（3）休克发生发展中的三个阶段微循环变化各有何特点？其产生机制及代偿意义是什么？

（4）以过敏性休克和感染性休克为例，探讨它们的发生机制各有何特点。救治时应采取哪些相应措施？

实验六 肠缺血再灌注损伤

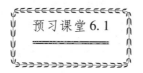

一、实验目的

（1）建立肠缺血再灌注损伤动物模型。

（2）观察肠缺血再灌注损伤的病理变化。

（3）探讨肠缺血再灌注损伤可能的发病机制。

二、实验原理

夹闭肠系膜上动脉一定时间会造成动物急性肠缺血，使肠黏膜屏障结构受到破坏，失去隔避肠内有毒物质进入循环的功能。此时若放开夹闭的肠系膜上动脉，恢复血流灌注，受损伤的肠黏膜屏障非但不会因为恢复血流灌注而恢复功能，反而会因为恢复血流灌注与供氧产生的氧自由基和钙超载而造成更严重的组织损伤，导致更多的肠内有毒物质进入循环，产生严重的毒血症，引起血压下降。

三、实验材料

1. 实验动物

家兔。

2. 材料

（1）仪器及器材：兔台；手术器械；注射器；针头；动脉夹；压力传感器；BioLab-410生物机能实验系统。

（2）试剂：3%戊巴比妥钠；1%普鲁卡因；肝素钠；生理盐水。

四、实验步骤

（1）对家兔耳缘静脉注射 3% 戊巴比妥钠 1 mL/只来进行基础麻醉，使其仰卧固定于兔台上。

（2）腹壁正中备皮，上腹正中用 1% 普鲁卡因进行局麻。

（3）从胸骨剑突下 5 cm 起，做上腹正中切口，长 15~20 cm，沿腹白线打开腹腔，将肠管推向左侧，暴露右肾和脊柱。以右肾为标志，沿脊柱和肠系膜根部寻找肠系膜上动脉，小心分离肠系膜上动脉，穿线备用。

（4）颈部正中备皮，局麻后分离一侧颈总动脉。

（5）耳缘静脉注射肝素钠（1 mL/只）后，行颈总动脉插管，记录正常动脉血压值。

（6）待动脉血压平稳后，用动脉夹夹闭肠系膜上动脉。根据实验需要确定夹闭时间，用盐水纱布覆盖腹部切口，并观察肠系膜上动脉夹闭期间动脉血压的变化。

（7）到规定的夹闭时间后开放动脉夹，恢复血流灌注。观察肠再灌注期间动脉血压的变化。

五、注意事项

（1）本实验不宜使用过量的戊巴比妥钠，以免影响血压观察。

（2）翻动肠子的动作要轻柔，避免过度牵拉肠管引起低血压。

（3）用动脉夹夹闭肠系膜上动脉必须牢固可靠。

（4）松夹后可能由于夹闭处动脉壁黏连不能恢复血流灌注，达不到再灌注的实验目标，可用手指轻搓动脉夹夹闭处松解之。

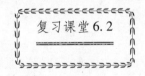

复习课堂 6.2

六、思考题

（1）通过分析实验结果，能得出什么结论？

（2）为什么肠缺血时血压变化不大，而再灌注会引起血压明显下降？

（3）为什么肠缺血不同时间后再灌注会引起不同的血压变化？

实验七　急性右心衰竭

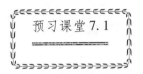

预习课堂7.1

一、实验目的

（1）复制急性肺小动脉栓塞及过量输液造成的家兔急性右心衰竭模型。

（2）观察急性右心衰竭时血流动力学改变并进行血气分析。

（3）探讨心功能发生变化的可能机理。

二、实验原理

心脏舒缩功能障碍和心脏负荷过重是心力衰竭的两大起因，后者又分为前负荷过重、后负荷过重。本实验用过量输液和栓塞肺小动脉的方法增加右心前、后负荷，并通过测量相应指标观察心功能变化，从而加深对心力衰竭发病机制的理解。此外，本实验还涉及缺氧、水肿、酸碱平衡紊乱等多个病理生理过程，通过对实验过程和实验数据的观察和分析，了解各个病理生理过程之间的相互联系。

三、实验材料

1. 实验动物

家兔。

2. 材料

（1）仪器与器材：兔台；手术器械一套；BioLab - 410 生物机能实验系统；血气分析仪；压力换能器；呼吸传感器；颈、股动脉套管；三通；注射器；小儿头皮针；输液装置；中心静脉压测量装置；听诊器。

（2）试剂：1% 普鲁卡因；3% 戊巴比妥钠；肝素钠注射液；肝素生理盐水溶液；生理盐水；液体石蜡。

四、实验步骤

（1）取家兔 1 只称重，经耳缘静脉注射 1 mL/kg 3% 戊巴比妥钠，将其麻醉后仰卧固定于兔台上。

（2）颈部及一侧腹股沟区备皮，用 3~5 mL 1% 普鲁卡因进行局麻。

（3）分离一侧颈总动脉和双侧颈静脉、一侧股动脉。分离气管并做气管插管。

（4）经耳缘静脉注射肝素钠 1 mL/只。

（5）将呼吸传感器与气管插管及 BioLab – 410 生物机能实验系统连接，记录呼吸频率和幅度。

（6）颈动脉插管（管内充满肝素生理盐水），通过压力换能器将其与 Bio-Lab – 410 生物机能实验系统连接。

（7）股动脉插管（管内充满肝素生理盐水），接三通注射器备采血供血气分析用。

（8）左侧颈静脉插管连接输液装置，以 10 滴/分钟速度输液。

（9）调节中心静脉压测量装置"0"位和家兔腋中线处于同一平面，连接中心静脉压测量装置的插管插入右侧颈静脉。插管过程可见中心静脉压测量装置液面不断降低，插入 5~6 cm 时，液面停止下降且随呼吸波动，该高度即为中心静脉压值，此时固定插管。

（10）观察动物一般状况，记录一段正常血压、呼吸曲线；听诊正常心音、呼吸音；测量中心静脉压和血气值；做肝—中心静脉压反流试验（轻推压右肋弓下 3 秒，中心静脉压上升的 cmH_2O 柱可表示之）。

（11）用小儿头皮针在耳缘静脉穿刺，用 1 mL 注射器取温度为 38 ℃ 液体石蜡经耳缘静脉以 0.1 mL/min 速度缓慢注入，同时密切观察。当动脉血压有明显下降或中心静脉压有明显上升时，即停止注射；如上述两指标又恢复到原对照水平，可再次缓慢注射液体石蜡，直至动脉血压下降 10~20 mmHg 或中心静脉压有明显上升为止（一般液体石蜡用量不超过 0.5 mL/kg）。用生理盐水保持耳缘静脉通畅。

（12）重复实验步骤（10）。

（13）5 分钟后，以每分钟 80 滴/分钟的速度快速经静脉输入生理盐水，同时观察测量上述各项指标并记录，直至家兔死亡。

（14）挤压胸壁观察：气管分泌物颜色、性状；剖开胸、腹，观察：有无胸、腹水；心脏及心腔体积；肺外观和肺切面；肝脏体积、外观。

（15）最后剪开腔静脉待血液流出后，观察心脏及肝体积改变。

五、注意事项

液体石蜡用量是成败的关键，过多、过快容易造成动物猝死，过少、过慢则效果不明显。当输液量超过 200 mL/kg，各项指标变化仍不显著时，可再次补注少量液体石蜡。

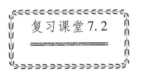

复习课堂 7.2

六、思考题

（1）本实验中有哪些指标可帮助判断急性右心衰竭的发生，为什么？

（2）为什么栓塞肺小动脉和过量输液可造成心脏负荷过重？

（3）动物死后解剖可观察到哪些异常变化，为什么会出现这些变化？

（4）心衰发生后，机体可能产生怎样的代偿反应？本实验中是否出现了这些反应？请解释为何有或无这些反应。

（5）中心静脉压的变化在心衰诊断治疗中有何意义？

（6）本实验还涉及缺氧、水肿、酸碱平衡紊乱等多个病理生理过程，它们是怎样发生的？相互间有何关系？

（7）心衰发生时血气分析结果会出现哪些变化？说明什么问题？

实验八　呼吸衰竭

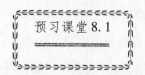

预习课堂 8.1

一、实验目的

（1）建立动物窒息、气胸及肺水肿模型。

（2）观察肺通气障碍、气体弥散障碍以及肺泡通气—血流比例失调引起的不同类型的呼吸衰竭。

二、实验原理

夹闭气道引起窒息，导致阻塞性通气障碍。而气胸对呼吸功能的影响主要取决于胸膜腔内气体的容量，注入少量气体造成轻度气胸时，则通气减少引起肺泡通气—血流比例失调；严重气胸时可造成严重的限制性通气障碍，总肺泡通气量显著减少，同时存在通气—血流比例失调，呼吸衰竭的主要机制是通气不足。弥散障碍及通气—血流比例失调则在肺水肿引起的呼吸衰竭机制中起主要作用。

三、实验材料

1. 实验动物

家兔。

2. 材料

（1）仪器及器材：兔台；BioLab–410 生物机能实验系统；手术器械一套；Y 形气管插管；注射器；50 mL 注射器（注射空气用）；7 号、16 号针头；三通；弹簧夹。

（2）试剂：1%普鲁卡因；3%戊巴比妥钠；20%葡萄糖溶液。

四、实验步骤

（1）对家兔经耳缘静脉注射3%戊巴比妥钠1 mL/只，使其仰卧，固定于兔台上。

（2）颈部正中备皮，注射3~5 mL 1%普鲁卡因来进行局麻，分离气管，在甲状软骨下0.5~1 cm处做"⊥"形切口（可酌情使用局麻），插入Y形气管插管。通过呼吸传感器使其连接BioLab-410生物机能实验系统，记录呼吸频率和深度。

（3）复制窒息：

①用弹簧夹将Y形气管插管上端橡皮管完全夹住，使动物处于完全窒息30秒，描记呼吸曲线。

②放开弹簧夹，等待5分钟，让动物恢复正常。重复3次。

（4）复制气胸：

①于家兔右胸第4~5肋间隙用16号针头穿刺（有明显突破感即进入胸腔），该针头用三通连接50 mL注射器。向胸腔内缓慢注入空气，30 mL/次，观察呼吸频率及幅度变化。若无改变，继续注入空气直至出现变化，并描记呼吸曲线。

②用50 mL注射器将胸腔内空气抽尽，拔出针头。

③观察10~20分钟，待动物呼吸恢复正常。

（5）复制肺水肿：

①将家兔头端兔台垫高，从Y形气管插管一侧缓慢滴注20%葡萄糖溶液（2 mL/次），观察呼吸频率及幅度。若无改变，继续滴注，直至出现呼吸变化，并描记呼吸曲线。

②出现明显的呼吸变化后夹住气管，处死家兔，打开胸腔，用线在气管分叉处结扎，以防止肺水肿液流出。在结扎处以上切断气管，小心将心脏及其血管分离，取出肺，用滤纸吸去肺表面的水分后称取肺重，计算肺系数。

$$肺系数 = \frac{肺重量（g）}{体重（kg）}$$

③切开肺脏，观察有无泡沫样液体流出。

五、注意事项

（1）气胸后胸腔内的空气一定要抽尽。

（2）复制肺水肿时，从 Y 形气管插管滴注葡萄糖溶液不能太快，以免造成窒息。

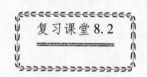

复习课堂 8.2

六、思考题

（1）窒息、肺水肿及气胸时的血气变化如何？

（2）窒息、肺水肿及气胸对呼吸有何影响？为什么？

（3）复制窒息后可将实验步骤中（1）（2）重复 2～3 次，能看到什么现象？为什么？

实验九 肝性脑病

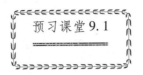

一、实验目的

（1）建立动物氨中毒模型。

（2）观察氨的毒性作用以及结扎大部分肝叶造成急性肝功能衰竭后动物对氨的敏感性变化，从而验证"肝性脑病"氨中毒学说，探讨氨中毒的可能机制。

二、实验原理

采用肝叶大部分结扎术，造成动物急性肝功能不全，在此基础上经十二指肠插管灌注氯化铵溶液，使实验动物血氨迅速升高，并出现抽搐、昏迷等类似肝性脑病的表现，证明氨在肝性脑病发病机制中的作用。另设立两对照组，其中一组动物在肝叶大部分结扎术后不输入氯化铵溶液，而代之以生理盐水，以证明"急性肝功能不全"因素在实验课期间尚不足以引发脑病；另一组动物不做肝叶大部分结扎术，而经十二指肠插管灌注氯化铵溶液，当输入量与肝叶大部分结扎术后灌注氯化铵溶液导致动物发病所需量相当时，动物不出现症状，表明肝具有对氨的解毒功能。

三、实验材料

1. 实验动物

家兔。

2. 材料

（1）仪器及器材：兔台；手术器械一套；注射器；针头；导尿管；粗棉

线；缝针。

（2）试剂：1%普鲁卡因；生理盐水；复方氯化铵溶液。

四、实验步骤

（1）取家兔一只（以下称甲兔），称重后使其仰卧固定于兔台上，腹壁正中备皮，在上腹正中用1%普鲁卡因进行局麻。

（2）从胸骨剑突起，做上腹正中切口，长8~10 cm，打开腹腔后，即可见位于右上腹的肝脏，向下挤压肝，剪断肝与横膈之间的镰状韧带，再将肝叶向上翻，用手剥离肝胃韧带。

（3）用粗棉线结扎肝左外叶、左中叶、右中叶和方形叶的根部（仅留下右外叶和尾状叶），使之血流阻断。

（4）沿胃幽门找出十二指肠，做荷包缝合。用眼科剪在荷包中央做一小切口，将导尿管向十二指肠远端空肠方向插入约5 cm，收紧荷包缝线以固定插管，再缝合腹壁。将导尿管固定在兔耳上。

（5）观察家兔的一般情况，如角膜反射及对疼痛刺激的反应。

（6）每隔5分钟向十二指肠插管中注入3 mL复方氯化铵溶液，观察动物的反应变化，直至痉挛发作为止，记录所用的复方氯化铵溶液总量。

（7）另取一只家兔（以下称乙兔），依次重复上述实验步骤（1）（2）（4）（5）（6）。该兔作为假手术对照组，除了不结扎肝叶外，其他所有操作与甲兔相同。

（8）再取一只家兔（以下称丙兔），依次重复上述实验步骤（1）（2）（3）（4）（5）。以后每隔5分钟向十二指肠插管中注入3 mL生理盐水，观察家兔有无异常变化。

五、注意事项

（1）剪断镰状韧带时，谨防刺破膈肌，造成气胸。在分离肝脏时，动作宜轻柔，以免肝叶破裂出血。

（2）结扎线应扎于肝叶根部，避免拦腰勒破肝脏。

（3）荷包缝合应选在十二指肠壁血管分布稀疏的部位进行。

（4）复方氯化铵溶液切勿漏入腹腔。

（5）复方氯化铵溶液配方：将 25 g 氯化铵、15 g 碳酸氢钠溶于 1 000 mL 5%葡萄糖溶液中。

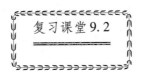

复习课堂 9.2

六、思考题

（1）通过分析实验结果，能得出什么结论？

（2）动物氨中毒为什么会引起神经系统功能障碍？

（3）单纯结扎大部分肝叶可否引起肝性脑病？为什么丙兔在实验课期间未出现明显症状？

（4）单纯灌注复方氯化铵溶液的乙兔，在复方氯化铵溶液输入量与甲兔发病所需量相当时，并不出现症状，为什么？如继续灌注复方氯化铵溶液，乙兔可否出现症状？为什么？

实验十　急性肾功能衰竭

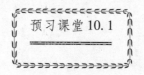

预习课堂 10.1

一、实验目的

（1）学习复制急性中毒性肾功能衰竭模型。

（2）观察实验动物血清、尿中钠和肌酐（Cr）含量的变化，理解急性肾功能衰竭的机能代谢变化。

二、实验原理

皮下或肌肉注射肾毒物氯化高汞（$HgCl_2$）溶液，会引起急性肾小管坏死，导致急性肾功能衰竭。

三、实验材料

1. 实验动物

家兔。

2. 材料

（1）仪器及器材：1 mL、5 mL 注射器；0.5 mL、2 mL、5 mL 刻度吸管；试管；滴管；玻璃棒；台式离心机；恒温水浴箱；721 型分光光度计。

（2）试剂：3% 焦锑酸钾溶液；无水乙醇；氢氧化钙；140 mmol/L 钠标准应用液；50 mmol/L 苦味酸溶液；pH 为 12.0 的磷酸盐—氢氧化钠缓冲液；2 mg% 肌酐标准应用液；1% 氯化高汞溶液；0.1% 肝素生理盐水。

四、实验步骤

（1）对家兔称重，实验前 24 小时经皮下或肌肉注射 1% 氯化高汞

（1.5～1.7 mL/kg），家兔放集尿笼内饲养，自由进食。

（2）收集 24 小时混合尿，并于注射氯化高汞 24 小时后心脏采血 3～5 mL，经 2 000 转/分钟离心 15 分钟，分离血清。

（3）应用焦锑酸钾比浊法测定钠含量。

①尿预处理：吸取 5 mL 尿液，移入含 0.2 g 氢氧化钙的试管中，用玻璃棒搅匀，放置 15 分钟，经 2 000 转/分钟离心 5 分钟，吸上清液放入另一试管内，此即尿滤液。

②钠含量测定方法见表 3-1。

表 3-1 钠含量测定方法

（单位：mL）

	空白管	标准管	血清测定管	尿液测定管
血清	—	—	0.2	—
尿滤液	—	—	—	0.2
钠标准液	—	0.2	—	—
蒸馏水	0.2	—	—	—
无水乙醇	1.8	1.8	1.8	1.8
混合后，离心（2 000 转/分钟×3 分钟），取上清液分别移入另一试管				
上清液	0.25	0.25	0.25	0.25
3% 焦锑酸钾溶液	5.0	5.0	5.0	5.0

混合后静置 5 分钟，使用 721 型分光光度计（520 nm 波长），以空白管调零，测定各管光密度值。

③计算：

$$钠浓度（mmol/L）= \frac{测定管光密度值}{标准管光密度值} \times 140$$

（4）应用苦味酸沉淀蛋白法测定肌酐含量。

①尿预处理：1∶50 稀释尿滤液。

②肌酐含量测定方法见表 3 - 2。

表 3 - 2　肌酐含量测定方法

（单位：mL）

	空白管	标准管	血清测定管	尿液测定管
血清	—	—	0.6	—
1：50 尿滤液	—	—	—	0.6
钠标准液	—	0.6	—	-
蒸馏水	0.6	—	—	-
50 mmol/L 苦味酸溶液	2.4	2.4	2.4	2.4
混合 3 分钟后，离心（2 000 转/分钟×10 分钟），取上清液分别直接倾入另一试管				
pH 为 12.0 磷酸盐—氢氧化钠缓冲液	0.6	0.6	0.6	0.6

充分混匀，置 37 ℃水浴箱中 25 分钟，冷却静置 20 分钟，使用 721 型分光光度计（525 nm 波长），以空白管调零，测定各管光密度值。

③计算：

$$肌酐浓度（mg/dL）= \frac{测定管光密度值}{标准管光密度值} \times 2$$

（5）取另一只正常家兔作对照，按上述方法测定血清、尿中钠和肌酐的含量。

五、实验结果记录

检测项目	正常兔	急性肾衰兔
尿钠		
血清钠		
尿肌酐		
血清肌酐		

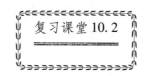

复习课堂 10.2

六、思考题

（1）引起急性肾功能衰竭的常见肾毒物有哪些？

（2）氯化高汞可引起什么类型的急性肾功能衰竭？

（3）氯化高汞会引起哪些肾组织结构的病变？其导致急性肾功能衰竭的机制是什么？

（4）急性肾功能衰竭可引起机体哪些机能代谢变化？

第四部分　临床病例讨论

【讨论一】

1. 患者女性，16 岁，糖尿病酮症入院。在急诊室呈昏迷状态，皮肤松弛，弹性差，眼窝凹陷，呼吸深快，血压 90/60 mmHg。

化验： 血清 Na^+ 151 mmol/L，血清 K^+ 3.6 mmol/L，血糖 453 mg%，血浆尿素氮（BUN）36 mg%，血 pH 7.2，血氧分压 27 mmHg，标准碳酸氢盐 16 mmol/L。

问题：

（1）患者有无水钠代谢紊乱？属何种类型？为什么？

（2）患者有无钾代谢紊乱？属何种类型？为什么？

（3）患者有无酸碱平衡紊乱？属何种类型？为什么？

（4）本病例应如何治疗？有何需要注意之处？

2. 患者男性，28 岁，因腹泻不能进食 3 天，在当地诊所服药补液后未见好转入院。患者精神萎靡，眼窝下陷，四肢静脉不显，呈明显脱水状，但口渴不明显，呼吸深，腹胀，四肢软弱无力，血压 80/60 mmHg。

化验： 血清 Na^+ 120 mmol/L，血清 K^+ 3.0 mmol/L，血 pH 7.32，标准碳酸氢盐 18 mmol/L，剩余碱 −5 mmol/L。

问题：

（1）患者有无水钠代谢紊乱？属何种类型？为什么？

（2）患者有无钾代谢紊乱？属何种类型？为什么？

（3）患者有无酸碱平衡紊乱？属何种类型？为什么？

（4）本病例应如何治疗？有何需注意之处？

3. 患者男性，56 岁，出现肺水肿入院。

化验：血气分析结果为 pH 7.22，HCO_3 20 mmol/L，血氧分压 50 mmHg。

问题：该患者发生了何种酸碱平衡紊乱？其依据是什么？

【讨论二】

1. 患者男性，30 岁。因发热、咳嗽和全身无力就诊。诊断为感冒，给予吗啉胍、扑热息痛、止咳剂治疗未见好转。39 ℃以上高热持续 10 天。

体检：体温 40.2 ℃，心率 90 次/分，呼吸 30 次/分，血压 126/86 mmHg。脾肿大。

化验：白细胞总数 $3.5 \times 10^9/L$，血培养发现伤寒杆菌。

患者经相应治疗后痊愈。

2. 患者男性，8 岁。因发热、恶心、烦躁不安而就诊入院。

体检：体温 39.3 ℃，心率 122 次/分，呼吸 32 次/分，血压 90/60 mmHg。

给予抗菌治疗，症状未见好转。患儿隔日定时出现寒战高热，体温高达 40.5 ℃。高热后全身出汗，体温迅速下降。经血检查出间日疟原虫。给予抗疟治疗后痊愈。

3. 患者女性，15 岁。因发热 36 天，全身关节肿痛 30 天，急诊入观察室。其间曾数次服用解热镇痛药和抗菌素，关节肿痛可缓解，但发热仍持续，基本未超过 39 ℃。

体检：体温 38 ℃，心率 120 次/分，呼吸 20 次/分，血压 110/76 mmHg。

化验：抗核抗体（ANA）1∶640，Smith 酸性核蛋白（SM）抗体阳性，总补体以及补体 C_3 均降低。

患者被诊断为系统性红斑狼疮（SLE），经给予激素和对症治疗后，病情缓解。

问题：

（1）发热这一病理过程可能出现在哪些疾病当中？

（2）上述病例中发热的热型、原因及机制是什么？

（3）发热三个时相体温变化的机制、热代谢特点是什么？

（4）临床在输液过程中出现发热首先应考虑什么？

（5）结合发热给机体带来的双重影响，临床在进行解热治疗时应注意哪些问题？

4. 患者女性，14 岁。1 天前她于游泳后出现发热，伴头痛、全身肌肉酸痛、食欲减退、轻咳无痰、呕吐胃内容物 1 次，无抽搐、腹痛等不适。门诊以"发热待查"收治入院。

体检：体温 39.7 ℃，脉搏 112 次/分，呼吸 28 次/分，血压 120/70 mmHg，神志清楚，精神差，急性热病容，全身未见皮疹及出血点，咽充血，双侧扁桃体肿大，可见少许脓栓，双侧颈部淋巴结肿大。心、肺检查未及异常。腹软，未及肝脾，无病理反射。尿少色黄。化验见白细胞计数 14.7×10^9/L，中性粒细胞比值 81.6%，淋巴细胞比值 11.7%。入院后给予抗生素及输液治疗。

在输液过程中出现畏寒、寒战、烦躁不安。体温升至 41 ℃，心率 128 次/分，呼吸浅促，立即停止输液，肌内注射异丙嗪 1 支，并给予乙醇擦浴，头部置冰袋。次日，体温渐降，患者精神萎靡，出汗较多，继续输液及抗生素治疗。3 天后，体温降至 37 ℃，除感乏力外，无自觉不适。住院 6 天痊愈出院。

问题：

（1）入院时的发热是什么引起的？本病可能的诊断是什么？

（2）输液过程中出现的畏寒、寒战、体温升高等属何种反应？为什么？

（3）给患者用乙醇擦浴、头部置冰袋处理的意义何在？

【讨论三】

患者女性，65 岁。有冠心病心绞痛病史 8 年，无高血压史，夜间突发心前区疼痛 8 小时入院。

体检： 入院时血压为 150/90 mmHg，经心电图检查，诊断为急性前壁心肌梗死。采用溶栓治疗后，心前区疼痛缓解。后出现心律失常，血压 70/50 mmHg，出冷汗，面色苍白，窦性心律，心率 126 次/分。

问题：

（1）患者出现心功能降低即心肌顿抑的表现，简述其发生机制。

（2）经冠状动脉造影诊断，患者部分心肌出现无复流现象，简述其可能机制。

（3）试述缺血—再灌注损伤时氧自由基生成过多的机制。

（4）试述氧自由基如何造成机体损伤。

（5）试述缺血—再灌注损伤时细胞内钙超载的发生机制。

（6）试述缺血—再灌注损伤的防治原则。

【讨论四】

患者女性，27 岁，因妊娠停经 40 周，破水 2 天，阵发性腹痛 12 小时，寒战 2 小时，于凌晨 1 时急诊入院。

患者停经 6 周时出现恶心呕吐等早孕反应，妊娠 20 周出现胎动，妊娠期间无阴道出血，未进行过定期产前检查。平常月经规律，无痛经史、闭经史。

体检：体温 38.2 ℃，呼吸 21 次/分，血压 110/70 mmHg，心率 86 次/分。心律齐，腹膨隆，宫底剑突下 3 cm，全腹压痛（＋），胎心为零。产科检查为内诊阴道通畅，充血，羊水 Ⅲ°、恶臭，宫口开大 7 cm。

化验：血常规为血红蛋白浓度 125 g/L，红细胞计数 4.2×10^{12}/L，白细胞计数 14.0×10^9/L，中性粒细胞比值 80%，淋巴细胞比值 20%。

治疗经过：入院经吸氧、静推小三联（5% 葡萄糖 ＋ 维生素 C ＋ 地塞米松）、安定治疗后，寒战停止，但胎心不恢复，仍诉腹痛。宫口开全时行胎吸，穿颅人工助产，分娩出一死婴，死婴全身皮肤斑片状剥脱，恶臭。产中产后出血约 200 mL，患者主诉腹痛不能耐受，面色青紫，阴道出血量不多。立即胸腹联透示肠管大量积气，无液平，返回病房时血压降至零，呼吸急促，面部青紫加重，神志蒙眬，血压不升，心率 140 次/分，心律不齐，腹腔穿刺抽出不凝血。疑为子宫破裂大出血，立即行剖腹探查，见子宫完整，收缩不良，肠系膜弥漫性渗血，胃肠严重肿胀，胃管行胃肠减压抽出血性胃内容物约 3 000 mL。术中快速输鲜血 2 000 mL，切除子宫关腹。血压波动在 90～70/60～40 mmHg，全身皮肤黏膜青紫进一步加深，伴大量斑片状出血，3P 试验阳性，意识蒙眬，双肺底可闻及湿啰音。经抗炎、输新鲜血、扩容升压等抢救治疗，于当天 13 时呼吸心跳停止，临床死亡。

问题：

（1）根据病史、实验室检查及临产表现，对患者应作出哪些诊断？其依据是什么？

（2）病程的演变过程是怎样的？

（3）患者为什么会出现腹痛、寒战、发热？

（4）患者为什么白细胞和中性粒细胞增多？

（5）患者为什么会出现血压降低？

（6）患者为什么会出现肠系膜弥漫性渗血、3P 试验阳性？

（7）患者为什么会出现双肺底可闻及湿啰音、胃肠严重肿胀？

【讨论五】

患者男性，27 岁，农民。因活动后心悸气促 4 月余，2 周来双下肢水肿伴有发热，加重 10 天入院。

现病史： 14 年前曾先后出现右膝关节、肩及左臂关节痛，但无红肿。2 年前再次发生右膝关节疼痛，伴有红肿及全身发热，经治疗（用药不详）而愈。4 个月前发觉每当活动后，即感心跳气短，同时经常咳嗽，有时痰中带血。3 个月前突然发生左上腹痛，2 天后消失。半月前开始双下肢上行性水肿，心悸气促加重，每于夜间平卧后即感气喘，胸闷难受，坐起后始觉好转。

体检： 体温 38 ℃，心率 130 次/分，呼吸 25 次/分，血压 120/80 mmHg。发育正常，营养中等，神志清，查体合作。半坐位。右上睑结膜有数个针头大小的出血点。口唇紫绀，双侧扁桃体Ⅰ度肿大。颈静脉怒张。心界扩大，心尖区可闻Ⅲ级收缩期吹风样杂音及舒张期隆隆样杂音，肺动脉瓣区第二音亢进，两肺可闻中小水泡音。腹部膨隆，肝大，在锁骨中线肋下 6 cm，剑突下 7 cm，硬度中等，有轻度压痛。脾在肋下 3 cm，双下肢凹陷性水肿，指端呈杵状。

化验： 痰中发现心力衰竭细胞，红细胞计数 330 万/mm^3，白细胞计数 10 600/mm^3，中性粒细胞比值 81%，淋巴细胞比值 17%；尿红细胞 4～5/高倍镜视野，尿蛋白（＋）。中心静脉压 19 cm H$_2$O，臂肺循环时间 12 秒。

治疗经过： 入院后给洋地黄制剂和利尿药，并用青霉素 80 万单位/日，链霉素 1 g/日，控制感染。入院后第 16 天出现右腰部疼痛，3 天后呼吸困难加重，烦躁不安，两肺布满大量水泡音，经应用西地兰及给氧等方法抢救无效，于当晚 10 时死亡。

尸检发现： 睑结膜有小出血点，口唇紫绀，杵状指。心脏体积增大，各心腔扩张，心室壁增厚，二尖瓣短缩增厚，变硬，根部互相粘连；腱索变短、粗而硬。主动脉瓣变厚短缩，根部互相粘连。心室内面可见灰褐色赘生物（有数个）。肺淤血，槟榔肝，脾和右肾有局灶性贫血性梗死。

问题：

（1）根据病史及尸检发现，对患者应作出哪些临床诊断？其根据是什么？

（2）本病的发病过程如何？（包括病因及发病机理）

（3）心尖区为什么能听到双期杂音？其产生的机理是什么？

（4）患者为什么出现咳嗽、气短、痰带血丝？为什么肺部可闻及中小水泡音及肺动脉瓣区第二音亢进？

（5）患者为什么夜间平卧后即感气喘、胸闷难受？又为什么坐起来始觉好转？

（6）患者为什么会出现中心静脉压升高？臂肺循环时间延长？

（7）患者为什么有颈静脉怒张、肝脾肿大？

（8）患者为什么出现双下肢凹陷性水肿？其产生机理是什么？

（9）患者为什么出现左上腹、右腰部疼痛？为什么会出现白细胞计数增多，其中性粒细胞比值为81%，还会出现红细胞计数减少？为什么尿红细胞（＋＋），尿蛋白（＋）？

（10）患者为什么发热？其发生机理是什么？

【讨论六】

患者男性，56 岁。因反复咳喘 13 年，双下肢浮肿 2 年，加重 3 天入院。

现病史： 患者于 13 年前患感冒、发热，出现咳喘，开始少量白色痰，后变黄痰，经治疗好转，但每于冬春季节或气候突变就会反复发作。之后他一直能参加农业劳动，但上述症状逐年加重。近 6 年来发作频繁，劳累后感心悸气促，休息后好转。近 2 年来出现下肢浮肿，腹胀。平时有轻咳喘，咳白色痰，夜间较重，多于晨 4~5 点出现喘息。3 天前因患感冒、发热，黄痰，咳喘加重，食欲差，少尿而入院。

体检： 神志清，自动体位，呼吸稍促，口唇轻度紫绀，伴面部水肿，颈静脉怒张，肝颈静脉回流征（+）。胸廓前后径增宽，肋间隙增宽。叩诊呈过清音，肺肝界于右第六肋间。双肺可闻及干湿啰音。心尖搏动不明显，心界无明显扩大，心音弱，各瓣膜区无明显杂音。心率 116 次/分，可闻期前收缩。腹软，右上腹压痛明显，肝大，在右肋下 2.5 cm，脾未触及，移动性浊音（+）。双下肢凹陷性水肿。

化验： 白细胞计数 9 800/mm^3，中性粒细胞比值 75%，淋巴细胞比值 25%，血氧分压 50 mmHg，HCO_3^- 27.3 mmol/L，标准碳酸氢盐 20.5 mmol/L，pH 7.1。肝功能正常，血清总蛋白 3.7 g/dL，其中白蛋白 2.4 g/dL，球蛋白 1.3 g/dL。

心电图检查： P 波高尖，顺钟向转位，右室肥厚，心肌劳损，多源性期前收缩。

X 线检查： 肺动脉段突出，右室增大，肺野透亮度增强，肺门纹理增粗。

治疗经过： 入院后经抗感染、祛痰、利尿、强心等治疗，病情好转。

问题：

（1）病程演变过程是怎样的？

（2）患者呼吸功能状态及发生原理是怎样的？

（3）患者心脏功能状态及发生原理是怎样的？

（4）患者气促、紫绀、水肿的发生原理是什么？

【讨论七】

患者男性，45 岁。因慢性无黄疸型肝炎 9 年，腹水及全身水肿 3 个月，使用利尿药和保肝药物治疗，突然出现昏迷 1 天急诊入院。

体检：体温 37.2 ℃，脉搏 62 次/分，呼吸 18 次/分，血压 80/60 mmHg。神志蒙眬，检查不合作，皮肤、巩膜轻度黄疸，肝脾触诊不满意，腹部移动性浊音阳性，双下肢有凹陷性水肿。

化验：血清总胆红素（STB）22.3 μmol/L，其中结合胆红素（CB）8.2 μmol/L；丙氨酸氨基转移酶（ALT）160 U，白蛋白 3.3 g/dL，血清钾 1.96 mmol/L，血清钠 118 mmol/L，血清氯 64 mmol/L。粪便黑色，潜血试验阳性。

超声波检查：肝上界在第 6 肋间，剑突下 4.5 cm，右肋下 1 cm。波形呈较密微波至稀疏低小波，略迟钝，出波衰减。

治疗经过：入院后经使用精氨酸、谷氨酸钠、左旋多巴、食醋保留灌肠、新霉素、纠正电解质平衡紊乱、利尿、输新鲜血等措施治疗无效，于 1 周后死亡。死亡时从口中流出血性分泌物。

问题：

（1）对患者的诊断是怎样的？属于哪一种类型？

（2）正确的病因和诱因是什么？简述其根据。

（3）本病例可能有哪些毒物参与了该病理过程的发生？

（4）患者为何出现腹水及全身水肿？

（5）什么原因引起患者血清钾、血清钠、血清氯降低？这些对中枢神经系统有何影响？

【讨论八】

患者女性，19 岁，学生，1999 年 9 月 3 日急诊入院。

主诉：近两个月精神不振，嗜睡；近两周呕吐，尿少，排尿有灼热感，面部浮肿。

现病史：患者曾于 9 年前出现尿频、尿急和排尿灼热感，持续 6 个月。此后上述症状消失，但体力逐渐下降，因而不能参加学校正常活动。5 年前出现"贫血"，曾进行多种抗贫血治疗，但疗效不好。不久又出现多尿，烦渴。3 年前尿内发现"蛋白"，在过去的 2 年里经常发生鼻衄。近 2 年明显消瘦，疲乏无力加重。1 年前左腰部间歇性疼痛 6 小时，右侧卧可部分缓解。继后连续 3 天出现呕吐，吐出物为食物，但无发热和寒战，无血尿，尿内未见结石。曾于 1998 年 11 月住院检查，当时血压 140/80 mmHg。

化验：红细胞比容 23%，血红蛋白 7.5 mg%，血尿素氮（BUN）117 mg%，血非蛋白氮（NPN）143 mg%，血肌酐 7.6 mg%，血清钙 7.9 mg%，血清磷 8.5 mg%，标准碳酸氢盐 20 mmol/L。尿比重固定在 1.006~1.010，肌酐清除率为 6.8 mL/min，酚红排泄试验（PSP）15 分钟 <2%，X 线显示全身骨质脱钙。

近半年来又出现运动性气短，同时发现血压升高至 160/110 mmHg，X 线及心电图显示左心室肥大。近两个月食欲不振，并时有恶心、呕吐及左耻骨支持续性钝痛。此后精神日渐不支，嗜睡。近一周因患"感冒"，上述症状加重，每天呕吐 3~4 次，大便时干时稀，未见脓血。尽管进水量正常，但尿量减少，并有排尿灼热感及面部浮肿。

过去病史：患者学龄前曾有反复发作的咽痛史。7 岁时患"风湿热"。同年，作扁桃体切除。

体查：患者极度衰弱，面色苍白，消瘦，精神萎靡，反应迟钝，但意识清楚。面部轻度水肿，皮肤黏膜未见出血点。体温 37.2 ℃，血压 150/115 mmHg，脉搏 96 次/分。心界向左扩大，心尖可闻吹风样收缩期杂音，肺部检查无病理性发现。腹软，肝脾未触及。左下腹有轻度压痛，双侧肾区轻度叩击痛。双下肢未见凹陷性水肿。无病理反射体征。

化验：

血红细胞计数 250 万/mm^3，血红蛋白 7.2 mg%，红细胞比容 21%；

血白细胞计数 9 200/mm^3，中性粒细胞比值 85%；

血清钠 116 mmol/L，血清钾 4.9 mmol/L，血清氯 77 mmol/L，标准碳酸氢盐 16 mmol/L；

血清磷 9.5 mg%，血清钙 8.2 mg%，血非蛋白氮 268 mg%，血肌酐 15.7 mg%；

尿比重固定在 1.008～1.010，酚红排泄试验 15 分钟为 0，尿蛋白（＋＋＋＋），尿中有多量脓细胞、白细胞及管型。

X 线显示全身骨质脱钙，未见病理性骨折。

入院后，虽经积极治疗，但病情仍继续恶化，曾多次发生鼻衄。至 9 月 21 日，血压升至 250/130 mmHg，血非蛋白氮为 284 mg%，标准碳酸氢盐下降为 8 mmol/L，并有几次癫痫样痉挛发作，渐进入昏迷，于 9 月 28 日死亡。

尸检发现：患者肾脏为晚期慢性肾盂肾炎并有急性发作改变。甲状旁腺增大，全身骨质普遍脱钙，骨质变软。左心室肥厚扩大，二尖瓣关闭不全。结肠黏膜有溃疡形成。右肺下叶呈支气管肺炎变化。

问题：

（1）该患者的临床诊断是什么？有何依据？

（2）简述该病例的病情发生发展经过。

（3）该患者有哪些主要表现？是怎样发生的？

后　记

　　本书编者为多年工作在教学一线的骨干教师，有较丰富的理论教学与实验教学经验。但由于编写时间仓促，书中难免有缺点和疏漏之处，恳请同道和读者不吝赐教和指正，以便我们今后进一步修订完善。本书经陆大祥教授、陈燕萍教授、王方教授和暴克尧的审阅修订，得到编写人员所在院校以及暨南大学出版社的大力支持和鼓励。暨南大学国际学院和医学院的学生们也在使用中提出了宝贵的意见，编者在此一并致以衷心的感谢！

编者

2022 年 3 月

Chapter 1　Introduction

1. The objective of laboratory experiments in pathophysiology

Pathophysiology is a compulsory subject in medical education. It deals mainly with the pathogenesis, focuses on the dynamic functions and metabolic changes in diseases, depicts the typical patterns and clarifies the nature of health disorders.

Pathophysiology is also a subject that emphasizes both theoretical and experimental studies. The related fields such as biochemistry, physiology, anatomy and pathology should be reviewed to understand the relationship between metabolic changes and illness development.

In order to investigate the pathogenesis of diseases, numerous experiments have been conducted, especially by using laboratory animals to perform the investigations that are not permitted on human. It is necessary to establish animal models to establish or mimic the human diseases, to carefully observe the disorders of body functions and metabolisms, and to test new therapies.

Most achievements of pathophysiology come from experimental researches. Therefore, proper laboratory practices are arranged in the schedule of pathophysiology study. The purpose of these studies is to provide an opportunity for medical students, who have little clinical experience, to practise, observe and discuss the mechanism of diseases personally, and finally to confirm the theory taught in the lecture and to obtain a good training for establishing their scientific and clinical thinking and working capacities. Through the observation and analysis of scientific phenomena, the collection and arrangement of experimental data and the writing of experimental reports, students can preliminarily master the basic operation methods of pathophysiological experiments. The experiments will strengthen the cultivation of students' scientific research quality, train their self-study ability, hands-on ability and written expression ability, develop innovative thinking, and finally enable students to establish a rigorous and realistic scientific style.

2. General instructions for laboratory work

(1) Read the instruction thoroughly for each laboratory experiment, understand the objectives, principles, methods and procedures of the laboratory work, and review the related lectures before coming to the laboratory.

(2) Arrive on time. Wear laboratory coat. Do not do anything unrelated to the laboratory work in the classroom.

(3) Take good care of the school properties. Comply with the laboratory regulations consciously. Follow the instruction to operate the equipment carefully. Save on all articles for experiment use. Report should be made to the instructor when any damage of equipment happens.

(4) Pay close attention to personal safety. Prevent electrical injury, fire disaster, pathogen and chemical contamination, intoxication and animal bite. In case of injury, seek medical assistance and notify your instructor immediately for the necessary first aid or further medical treatment.

(5) Observe and record experimental results accurately and objectively. Revising and modifying any original data are strictly prohibited.

(6) Participating in lab discussion is strongly encouraged. Be prepared,

make standpoints clear-cut and full of grounds for argument in your speaking.

(7) Return all equipments and supplies to their appropriate places when the experiment is completed. Clean the lab bench and the classroom before leaving.

(8) Finish your laboratory report in a scientific manner and hand it over to your instructor for mark on time.

3. Requirements for laboratory reports

Writing laboratory reports is an important basic skill, which should be finished independently in a scientific manner: normative format, precise expression, objective description, reasonable discussion and analysis. A good report usually shows an author's reasoning, scientific thinking and his own opinion. Aimless transcription from the textbook should be avoided. Copying from others is a un acceptable behavior.

Please follow the format shown below:

(1) Name, grade, class and group.

(2) Project and date.

(3) Objectives and principles.

(4) Experimental subjects.

(5) Materials and methods.

(6) Results: Explain the pathophysiological effects of the experimental subject under the action of treatment factors. Detailed description can be explained in words. Charts can be used to list the experimental data after sorting out, and illustrated in words, so the result is clear and comparable.

(7) Discussion: According to the results of the experiment, explain and analyze the pathogenesis and theoretical basis. Analyze the causes of unexpected results in the experiment if there are any. The analysis and reasoning should be realistic, scientific and logical.

(8) Conclusion: The conclusion should be in accordance with the purpose of the experiment. It should be a general summary and judgment concluded from the experimental results and a concise summary of the theory that can be verified by the experiment.

Chapter 2　Laboratory Animals

1　Standardization and selection of laboratory animals

1.1　Superiority of using laboratory animals

Using laboratory animals makes things easy when researchers lay out control, design the experiment conditions, emphasize the treatment factor and avoid the interference of artifacts. The use of standardized experimental animals can carry out observations that cannot be done on human. By copying animal models of human diseases, large-scale studies can be carried out to overcome the limitations of sources and thus speed up the research process.

1.2　Limitation of using laboratory animals

The differences between human beings and laboratory animals include anatomic structures, physiological functions, metabolisms and sensitivity or reactivity to pathogens and drugs. Therefore, a conclusion from animal experiments should be carefully made and not be simply extended to humans. The effects of social and psychological factors on humans are difficult to be replicated on animals.

1.3　Standardization of laboratory animals

Standardization of laboratory animals means that the laboratory animals have the identification of their genetic background and degree of microbial cleaning. The animals are artificial breeding by strict procedures. Based on the genetic background, standard animals are divided into inbred strain animals, hybrid animals, closed colony animals and mongrel animals. According to the degree of microbial cleaning, the standard animals are divided into germ-free animals, gnotobiotic animals, specific pathogen-free animals, clean animals, and conventional animals.

1. 4　Selection of laboratory animals

There are a great variety of laboratory animals. The following tips can be used for your reference:

(1) Select the animals that are close to humans in anatomic structures, physiological functions, metabolisms and sensitivity or reactivity to pathogens and drugs.

(2) Select the animals that have a highly developed or specialized function, or a reactivity that is extremely sensitive, or an anatomic structure that is extraordinary convenient to observe in experiments.

In addition, select the animals with right age, sex, body weight to match your experimental needs. Pay close attention to the health condition of the animals. Be aware of the effects of seasons and biorhythms on your experiment results.

2　Drug administration and anesthesia of laboratory animals

2. 1　Route and method of drug administration in experimental animals

1. Intraperitoneal injection in mice

Hold the mouse with left hand, turn its head down and the abdomen up. Take the syringe in the right hand, insert the needle into the abdominal cavity from the left lower abdomen (avoid damaging the liver) to pierce the needle head at 45°,

2 – 3 mm deep. When there is no blood, intestinal juice or urine withdrawn, injection can be taken.

2. Intravenous injection of drugs at ear margin of rabbits

First, place the rabbit in the holding box. Before injection, the hair at the injection site should be removed, and gently flip the rabbit's ear with the finger to make the vein fill and expand. The index finger and middle finger of the left hand gently press the ear, while the thumb and ring finger fix the distal end of the auricular vein, and place the ring finger of the left hand under it as a cushion. After the vein is significantly filled, hold the syringe in the right hand, stab into the distal end of the vein, push 1 cm along the parallel direction of the blood vessel, and then relieve the pressure on the blood vessels at the root of the ear. Move the left thumb to fix the needle, and inject the drug liquid slowly. After injection, pull out the needle and press the needle hole with a dry cotton ball until no bleeding occurs.

2.2　Anesthesia of laboratory animals

In acute and chronic animal experiments, animals should be anesthetized before surgery, that is using specific drugs to inhibit the central nervous system to reduce or eliminate the pain of animals, make them quiet to ensure that the experiment is carried out smoothly. The anesthesia methods include general anesthesia and local anesthesia. The former one can be further divided into inhalation anesthesia and injection anesthesia. Injection anesthesia is mainly used in pathophysiological experiments.

1. General anesthesia

General anesthetics are mainly ethyl carbamate (urethane), sodium pentobarbital, chloral hydrate and so on. Injection anesthesia is usually administered intravenously or intraperitoneally. For intraperitoneal anesthesia, the total amount of anesthetic is usually injected in one go. Intravenous anesthesia works fast and its excitability period is short. The injection speed and quantity can be adjusted according to the reaction of experimental animals at any time, and it is easy to accurately reach the depth of anesthesia, so it is one of the most commonly used anesthesia methods.

(1) Mice: intraperitoneal injection with 30 – 90 mg/ (kg · BW) sodium pentobarbital.

(2) Rabbits: intravenous injection with 5 mL/ (kg · BW) 25% urethane.

2. Local anesthesia

For local anesthesia, intradermal injection or subcutaneous tissue infiltration injection is given at the surgical site with 1% procaine solution, which is mainly used to keep the animal awake and reduce pain.

3. Evaluation of anesthesia effect

The anesthetic effect of laboratory animals can be evaluated by visual observation or stimulus response.

(1) Complete anesthesia: After anesthetic is completely injected, the experimental animal's body naturally falls down, and its breathing becomes deep and slow, and the pupil is narrowed to 1/4 of the original, while the corneal reflex is dull, and the muscles of the limbs are relaxed, which shows the best anesthesia effect.

(2) Overdose of anesthetic: When an anesthetic overdose occurs, the animal either stops breathing and its heart stops beating, or the animal is bluish all over and its breathing is shallow and slow.

(3) Insufficient dose of anesthetic: If the animal is still struggling, screaming, sensitive to pain and breathing fast after injection, it should be observed for a period of time. If it is confirmed that the required depth of anesthesia is not reached, additional dose can be added again, which should not exceed 1/5 of the total amount at one time.

3　The use of common surgical instruments

Surgical instruments used in animal experiments are divided into general surgical instruments and microsurgical instruments. In this section, the correct holding and using method of common surgical instruments will be introduced.

3.1 Scalpel

The scalpel, composed of a knife handle and a blade, is mainly used to cut skin, tissue or organs and so on. Scalpels of different sizes and shapes can be selected according to different surgical sites and properties. Scalpel holding methods mainly include reverse pick type, holding type, pen type and bow type. When loading the blade, use the needle holder to hold the back of the front end of the blade, align the notch of the blade with the edge of the knife handle, and pull it back with a little force to install it. Similarly, to remove it, use a needle holder to hold the back of the end of the blade, extract the blade with a little force and push it forward.

When passing the scalpel, the passer should hold the back of the joint between the handle and the blade, and send the end of the handle to the operator's hands. Do not pass the blade straight to the operator, so as to avoid injury.

3.2 Scissors

Scissors are pointed or blunt, straight or curved and long or short.

1. Surgical scissors are used to cut nerves, human epidermal tissues or soft tissues.

2. Tissue scissors are used for cutting tissues. Most are curved scissors, sharp and fine, used to dissect, cut or separate tissues. Generally, straight scissors are suitable for the shallow operations; curved scissors are suitable for deep operations.

3. Thread scissors are used for cutting and removing sutures. Most are straight scissors. The difference between thread scissors and tissue scissors is that the blade of tissue scissors is sharp and thin, and the blade of thread scissors is blunt and thick. Therefore, thread scissors cannot be replaced by tissue scissors, so as to a-

void damaging to the blade.

4. Ophthalmic scissors are used to cut small soft tissues or nerves and blood vessels. Do not use ophthalmic scissors to cut hard materials such as skin, thread, gauze and so on, to avoid damaging the blade.

Correct holding method: When using scissors, insert the thumb and ring finger into the two rings of the handle, place the middle finger on the front handle, and use the index finger to press lightly on the shaft section. The thumb, middle finger and ring finger commonly control the opening and closing movements of the scissors, and the index finger is used to stabilize and control the direction of the scissors.

3.3　Surgical forceps

Commonly used surgical forceps are tooth forceps, smooth forceps and ophthalmic forceps. There are claw-shaped pinions that can bite each other on the head of the tooth forceps, which are used for clamping hard tissue from falling off. Smooth forceps, also called anatomical forceps, with a blunt, thick and smooth head as well as strips inside, can be used to clamp nerves, blood vessels, intestinal wall and other fragile tissues. Ophthalmic forceps are only used to clamp and separate fine tissues.

Correct holding method: Hold the middle part of the forceps with thumb, index finger and middle finger, clamp the tissue firmly and moderately.

3.4　Hemostatic forceps

1. Straight hemostatic forceps are used to separate superficial tissues and clamp bleeding blood vessels. Tooth hemostatic forceps are used to stop bleeding of tough tissues, lift skin and so on, but cannot be used for subcutaneous hemostasis.

2. Curved hemostatic forceps are mostly used for deep hemostatic surgery, and should not be used for nerves and other fragile tissues, so as to avoid unnecessary damage.

3. Mosquito hemostatic forceps are often used for delicate operations or small bleeding points, but not suitable for clamping large or hard tissues.

The method of holding hemostatic forceps is the same as that of surgical scissors. When opening, hold one ring of the hemostatic forceps with thumb and index finger, and hold the other ring with middle and ring finger. Gently push the thumb and ring finger against each other and immediately open the hemostatic forceps.

3.5 Needle holder

It is specially used for holding needles to stitch. Its shape is similar to the hemostatic forceps, but there is a short alveolar and a groove inside the head of needle holder generally.

3.6 Needles and sutures

Needles and sutures are used for suturing various tissues. There are round needles and three-edged needles, and for each type there are also curved and straight ones. The round needle is less traumatic, and usually used for soft tissues. The three-edged needle is often used for suture of skin and hard tissues. When using needle holder, it is advised to clamp the posterior 1/3 of the needle.

3.7 Arterial clamp

It is used to block arterial blood flow.

4   Basic surgical procedures

4.1 Skin preparation

After the animal is anesthetized, the site and scope of skin preparation should be determined, and the scope of skin preparation should be larger than the length of surgical incision. Commonly used methods for preparing skin are shearing and pluc-king.

1. Shearing

Tighten the skin of the surgical site, hold the curved surgical scissors flatly on the animal's skin with the right hand, and cut the hair against the direction. Do not lift the coat hair with hands when shearing, so as to avoid cutting the skin. Soak the clipped hair in water immediately to prevent the hair flying around.

2. Plucking

During intravenous injection of rabbit ears, use the thumb to pull out the hair of the desired experimental site gently.

4.2 Skin incision

1. Cut

Hold the hemostatic forceps with the left hand to lift the skin on one side of the pre-cut position, lift the corresponding skin on the opposite side with the help of an assistant. Then make a cut between the lifted skin to the required surgical incision length. When cutting the skin, avoid blood vessels.

2. Incision

The location, size and depth of the surgical incision should be determined by experimental requirements. Before cutting the tissue, use the fingers of left hand to pull the skin at the predetermined incision and make it tight. Use the scalpel to insert into the skin vertically, then move the scalpel at 45° with proper force, it would be best to cut the entire layer at one time. Cut the tissues layer by layer, and pay attention to hemostasis. Try as you might to make the direction of the incision consistent with the direction of the fibers of each tissue layer below the incision. The site of tissue incision should be preferentially selected where no important blood vessels or nerves sparseness. Avoid cutting blood vessels and nerves which may cause severe consequences.

4.3　Tissue separation

1.　Sharp dissection

Sharp dissection is using scissors, scalpel or other sharp instruments for delicate dissection and separation of skin, mucous membranes and dense tissues.

2.　Blunt dissection

Blunt dissection is often used to separate loose connective tissue between muscle and fascia by hemostatic forceps or fingers, etc. Soft tissues separation is mainly blunt dissection in principle, as they require to be separated layer by layer to keep the surgical field clear. Blood vessels should be avoided as well.

4.4　Hemostasis

Bleeding should be stopped immediately during the operation to prevent continued blood loss and maintain a clear surgical field. Commonly used hemostasis methods are compression hemostasis, clamp hemostasis and ligation hemostasis. Compression hemostasis is mostly suitable for capillary oozing blood. Press the bleeding site with a warm gauze. Clamp hemostasis is used to stop bleeding from small blood vessels. For large blood vessel bleeding, ligation hemostasis is often used. Clamp the bleeding site with hemostatic forceps first, and then ligate with silk thread (Note: be sure to tighten the knot to avoid false knots). If there is a lot of bleeding, use warm gauze to absorb the blood, then locate the bleeding site and clamp it with hemostatic forceps. Clamp the bleeding vessel wall accurately, avoid clamping the tissue around the blood vessel and do not clamp a large piece of tissue.

4.5　Basic surgery

Taking rabbits as experimental subjects, the basic surgical procedures are explained as follows:

1.　Tracheal separation and intubation

Make sure the rabbit is anesthetized, fixed and skin prepared. Make a 5 – 7 cm incision between the thyroid cartilage and the sternum along the midline of the neck with a scalpel to expose the sternohyoid muscle. Hemostatic forceps are then inserted along the midline into the left and right sternohyoid muscles for blunt dissection. Pull the left and right sternohyoid muscles laterally to expose the trachea. Below the larynx, use a curved hemostatic forcep to separate the trachea from the connective tissue behind it and thread a thick cotton thread. Pick up the cotton thread, cut the anterior segment of trachea horizontally between the two cartilage rings 2 cm below the thyroid cartilage with scissors (accounting for 1/3 – 1/2 of the wall of trachea), and make a 0.5 cm longitudinal incision towards the head to make it in the shape of "inverted T". Then the tracheal intubation tube is inserted into the tracheal cavity from the incision to the heart, ligated with the spare thread, and fixed the ligated thread to the "Y" type endotracheal intubation bifurcation to prevent the intubation from coming out. After insertion, check the tube for bleeding to keep airway smooth.

2. Common carotid artery separation and intubation

The purpose of common carotid artery intubation is to measure arterial blood pressure or for bloodletting use.

First, expose trachea of the rabbit following the steps above. The common carotid artery is located on both sides of the trachea. When separating, use hemostatic forceps to separate the connective tissue between the sternohyoid muscle and the sternothyroid muscle (i. e. in the Y-shaped groove) along the anterior edge of the sternal mastoid muscle. A large pink blood vessel can be found under the muscle suture, which has a throb feeling when touched by hand, namely the common carotid artery. The blood sheath is gently wiped with a cotton ball soaked in normal saline along the direction of the blood vessels. The common carotid artery is separated 2 – 3 cm along the direction of the blood vessels, and two silk threads soaked in normal saline are threaded under it for use. The surgical site should be kept moist and the blood should be wiped away during the procedure.

The distal end of the common carotid artery is ligated, and the artery is clamped to the proximal end with an arterial clamp. A V-shaped incision (about 1/3 of the diameter of the catheter) at 45° to the blood vessel is cut with ophthalmic scissors slightly near below the ligation point at the distal end, and then the catheter is fixed again with a thin thread at the distal end.

Note: Before arterial catheterization, the catheter is filled with 0.3% heparin sodium solution and the tee is closed at 45°.

3. External jugular vein separation and intubation

The purpose of external jugular vein intubation is for injection, blood collection, fluid infusion and central venous pressure measurement.

The external jugular vein is shallow and lies beneath the neck. After anesthesia, the rabbit is fixed in supine position, and the skin is cut a 6 – 8 cm incision in the middle. One side of the skin is lifted with the operator's left thumb and index finger, and the other fingers push up from the outside of the skin, then the skin is evaginated to reveal the dark purple thick blood vessel—external jugular vein. Gently separate the connective tissue around the vein with blunt hemostatic forceps along the direction of the blood vessel (do not pull too much during the separation process, and prevent to use scalpels or surgical scissors for separation, in order to avoid blood vessel rupture). The separation length is about 2.0 cm, and then leave two silk threads soaked with normal saline for use.

Before intubation, prepare the catheter, insert the end of a cut bevel, the other end is connected to the infusion device with normal saline, let the catheter filled with solution. The method of intubation is similar to that of the common carotid artery. For simple infusion, the length of the catheter into the blood vessel is generally 2 – 3 cm in rabbits. If the central venous pressure is measured, 5 cm should be inserted, and the catheter port is near the entrance of the superior vena cava close to the right atrium.

4. Femoral artery separation and intubation

The purpose of femoral artery separation and intubation is to separate femoral artery and vein, and to intubate femoral artery and vein for bloodletting, blood transfusion, infusion and drug injection. The femoral artery, femoral vein and femoral nerve lie beneath a layer of fascia and skin of the femoral triangle region of the medial side of the hind limb.

The procedures for femoral artery separation and intubation are as follows: after anesthesia, the rabbit is fixed in supine position, and the hair is clipped in the femoral triangle region for skin preparation. Touch the pulse of the femoral artery with hands, and make a 3 – 5 cm long skin incision along the direction of the artery. By blunt dissection of subcutaneous tissue and fascia with hemostatic forceps, femoral arteries, femoral veins and femoral nerves can be seen. The femoral vein is located on the inside, the femoral nerve is on the outside, and the femoral artery is located slightly behind the middle, just covered by the femoral nerve and femoral vein.

First, use mosquito forceps to separate the femoral nerve carefully, and then bluntly separate the connective tissue between the femoral artery and the femoral vein (Be careful not to damage the small branches of the blood vessel). The femoral artery segment is separated with a length of 2 – 3 cm, and 2 thin threads infiltrated by normal saline are inserted under it for use. The method of intubation is the same as that of the neck vessels.

Chapter 3　Experiments in Pathophysiology

Experiment 1　Factors Affecting Hypoxia Tolerance

1　Objectives

To understand the important role of factors involved in the pathogenesis of hypoxia, this experiment performs by altering the functional state of the central nervous system (CNS), the body metabolism and the ambient temperature.

2　Principles

In addition to the immediate causes of disease, there are various factors involved in the onset and development of diseases. Not only the extent and the rate of hypoxia, but also a number of factors, such as sex, biological rhythm, body metabolism, CNS function and ambient temperature, affect the hypoxia tolerance of the body. Among them, some may enhance the hypoxia tolerance, while the others may diminish it. In order to understand the role of these factors in causing disease, the effects of ambient temperature, body metabolism and the CNS function on the hypoxia tolerance to the mice which are hypotonic hypoxia are observed in this experiment.

3   Experimental materials

3.1   Animal

Mice.

3.2   Apparatus

Airtight bottle, clamp, apparatus for measuring oxygen consumption (Fig. 2), scales, 1 mL syringe, forceps, thermostatic water bath and mug.

3.3   Reagents

Soda lime, ice, normal saline (NS), 0.7% pentobarbital sodium, 4 mg/100 mL isoprenaline + 1 g/100 mL coramine solution.

4   Procedures

4.1   Hypoxia tolerance affected by different ambient temperatures

1. Place a bag of soda lime (about 5 g) into each of the three airtight bottles, respectively.

2. Select three mice with similar body weight, put them into the three airtight bottles respectively and label the bottles as A, B and C. Bottle A is immersed in ice water, bottle B is immersed in warm water (40 ℃ – 42 ℃) and bottle C is placed at room temperature. Tighten each bottle and clamp up the rubber tube.

3. Observe the activities and breathing behavior of the mice in the bottles and record their survival time. Remove the bottles from ice or warm water as soon as the mice is dead. After the bottles have been put at room temperature for 15 min, con-

nect the bottles to an apparatus for measuring the oxygen consumption of the mice.

4. Calculate the oxygen consumption rate (R) according to the following equation, where W is the weight of mice, t is the survival time and A is the total amount of oxygen consumption.

$$R \ (\text{mL/g} \cdot \text{min}) = \frac{A \ (\text{mL})}{W \ (\text{g}) \cdot t \ (\text{min})}$$

4.2 Hypoxia tolerance affected by different state of body function

1. Place a bag of soda lime into each of the three airtight bottles, respectively.

2. Select three mice with similar body weight. The mice are injected intraperitoneally with 0.1 mL/10 g of 4 mg/100 mL isoprenaline + 1 g/100 mL coramine solution, 0.1 mL/10 g of 0.7% pentobarbital sodium and 0.1 mL/10 g of normal saline, respectively.

3. Five minutes after injection, place the mice into three airtight bottles respectively, and clamp up the rubber tubes.

4. Observe the behavior of the mice in the bottles until they die, record the survival time.

5. Measure the oxygen consumption and calculate the oxygen consumption rate (R) of each mouse as described in section 4 of 4.1.

5 Cautions

1. Make sure the airtight bottles are airtight. If necessary, inject water to the interspace between the bottle and rubber stopper, the glass tube and the rubber stopper.

2. Make the intraperitoneal injection accurately on the left side of the abdomen

to avoid liver injury.

3. Determine the oxygen consumption by reading the falling level of water in graduated cylinder of the measuring apparatus.

6 Questions

1. What is the cause of death of mice during the experiment?

2. State the factors affecting hypoxia tolerance, and explain how they work.

APPENDIX I : Apparatus for measuring oxygen consumption

1 Principle

The mice in airtight bottle inhales the oxygen continuously, while the CO_2 exhaled is absorbed by soda lime, the equation is indicated as below:

$$NaOH \cdot CaO + H_2O + CO_2 \longrightarrow NaHCO_3 + Ca\ (OH)_2$$

As a result, the pressure in the bottle becomes negative, leading to the rise of water in the graduated pipette and the fall of water in the graduated cylinder when the bottle is connected to the measuring apparatus. The volume of the falling water equates to the total amount of oxygen consumption.

2 Methods

1. Pour water into the graduated cylinder to the maximal mark and connect the measuring apparatus to the airtight bottle with rubber tube as shown by Fig. 2.

2. Remove the clamp on the rubber tube. When the water in the pipette remains stable, the falling volume read from the graduated cylinder is equal to the total amount of oxygen consumed by the mice in the bottle.

APPENDIX II : Table for data collection

Group		Treatment	Weight W (g)	Survival time t (min)	Oxygen consumption A (mL)	Rate of oxygen consumption R (mL/g · min)
NO. 1	A	Ice water				
	B	40 ℃ – 42 ℃				
	C	Room temperature				
NO. 2	A_1	Isoprenaline + coramine solution				
	B_1	Pentobarbital sodium				
	C_1	Normal saline				

Experiment 2　Hyperkalemia

1　Objectives

1. Establish the animal model of hyperkalemia.

2. Observe the toxicity of hyperkalemia to rabbit heart.

3. Grasp the characteristic of electrocardiogram（ECG）changes in hyperkalemia.

4. Understand the principles of therapeutic strategy for hyperkalemia.

2　Principles

Serum potassium level in rabbit rises artificially（serum potassium concentration >5.5 mmol/L）after intravenous injection of potassium chloride. At the same time, by observing the changes of ECG on rabbit before and after the injection, we understand the toxic effects of hyperkalemia on the heart and the therapeutic treatments for rescuing arrhythmia（even cardiac arrest）induced by hyperkalemia are also performed with this animal model.

3　Experimental materials

3.1　Animal

Rabbit.

3.2　Apparatus

Electrocardiograph, hypodermic needle, syringe, rabbit holder.

3.3   Reagents

3% pentobarbital sodium, heparin sodium injection, potassium chloride solution at concentrations of 1%, 0.1% heparinized saline, etc.

4   Procedures

1. Weigh the rabbit. Inject 3% pentobarbital sodium at dose of 1 mL/kg intravenously in the marginal ear vein of the rabbit to make a general anesthesia. Then fix the rabbit in supine position with the rabbit holder.

2. Stick a needle electrode subcutaneously into the ankle: ***RED***—right forelimb, ***YELLOW***—left forelimb, ***BLACK***—right hindlimb and ***GREEN***—left hindlimb (Fig. 3).

3. Systemic heparinization is performed by intravenous injection of 1 mL of heparin sodium injection (12 500 U/2 mL) through the ear margin.

4. Connect the hypodermic needle to the syringe. Get rid of any air bubbles in the tubing. Insert the hypodermic needle into the marginal ear vein of the rabbit and fix it on the pinna of the ear securely with sticky tape. Adjust the transfusion rate to < 10 drops/min.

5. Turn on the electrocardiograph, select Lead II or avF to record the normal electrocardiogram for 3 – 4 heartbeats.

6. Begin at low dose, speed up the transfusion rate of 1% KCl in NS to 50 – 60 drops/min according to the physical state of the rabbit. Record the electrocardiogram with intervals of 3 minutes until the typical electrocardiogram of hyperkalemia is observed.

7. Maintain the transfusion rate of 1% KCl, record the electrocardiogram with intervals of 3 minutes until the rabbit dies. Pay close attention to the changes of electrocardiogram during the transfusion.

8. Dissect the rabbit, open the thorax and observe the situation of cardiac arrest.

5 Cautions

1. Inject pentobarbital sodium slowly to avoid the death of the animal.

2. Tolerance to the toxicity of potassium chloride solution varies individually. Some animals need higher doses than others to produce abnormal changes in their ECG.

3. The injection of potassium chloride solution should not be too fast, especially in the injection of high concentration, fast-speed will easily cause cardiac depression and death of the experimental animals, so that the typical ECG cannot be observed.

4. The injection should start from the distal end. If the ear vein cannot be injected because of repeated pierces, inject by the femoral vein.

5. The inner wall of hypodermic needle and syringe should be heparinized to prevent clotting.

6. Wipe with alcohol or normal saline after a needle electrode is used and remove the blood and water traces around electrodes and wires to maintain a good conductive state.

7. When tracing the ECG, pay attention to avoiding the surrounding electromagnetic interference and prevent the animals from struggling. If the animals struggle too frequently, add anesthetics through the ear vein, and start recording after they are stable, so as to prevent damage to the ECG machine.

6 Questions

1. What are the effects of hyperkalemia on cardiac functions?

2. What abnormal electrocardiogram have you seen during hyperkalemia? Try to explain the electrophysiological mechanism.

3. At the end of ventricular fibrillation, is it diastolic or systolic when you open the thorax? Why is that?

APPENDIX Ⅲ : Guide to use of electrocardiograph

1. Make sure the grounding cord of ECG machine (Fig. 4) is well connected before pressing the button "**POWER**".

2. Set the touch button "**PROG**" on the panel to "**MANUAL STD**", then set the chart speed at "**25**" (25 mm/s), voltage at "**10**" (0. 1 mV/ quadrate shelf).

3. Open "**HF**" (high frequency filter) and "**DF**" (drift filter), close "**MF**" (myoelectric filter).

4. Press "**PROG**" to select "**MANUAL STD**", choose " **Ⅱ** " or "**avF**".

5. Press "**RUN/STOP**" to record electrocardiogram. Press "**RUN/STOP**" again to stop recording.

Experiment 3　Fever

1　Objectives

1. Establish the fever models induced by endotoxin and endogenous pyrogen (EP).

2. Observe the changes of body temperature in response to endotoxin and EP.

3. Observe the thermotolerances of endotoxin and EP.

2　Principles

Endotoxin is a constituent of the outer cell wall of gram-negative bacteria. The active moiety of endotoxin is lipopolysaccharide (LPS). It's heat-resistant but can be inactivated by heating at 160 ℃ for 2 h. Endotoxin as an activator enters the body and activates cells capable of producing EP, then these cells produce and release EP, which makes the set-point of the hypothalamic thermostat shift upward, resulting in febrile response. Exdotoxin (0.5 μg/kg) causes a typical biphasic fever in rabbits. The first peak is at about 1 h after injection of endotoxin, and the second peak appears in about 3 h. Between the first and the second peak, a fall in body temperature is observed. The duration of febrile response induced by endotoxin is about 6 h.

EP is a heat-labile molecule and can be inactivated by heating at 90 ℃ for 30 min. The incubation period and duration of febrile response induced by EP are shorter than those by endotoxin. A regular dose of EP induces a monophasic fever while a very large dose of EP (40 mL/kg) may produce a biphasic fever.

3   Experimental materials

3.1   Animal

Rabbit weighing 2.0 – 3.0 kg.

3.2   Apparatus

Baby scale, electronic thermometer, febrile recording chart, thermostatic water bath, syringe, No.7 needle.

3.3   Reagents

Liquid paraffin, pyrogen-free normal saline (NS), endotoxin (0.2 μg/kg) in NS, EP solution.

4   Procedures

1. Weigh five healthy adapted rabbits and mark them as A, B, C, D and E.

2. Insert a thermistor probe into the rectum of each of the rabbits. Monitor the rectal temperature at least 3 times in 10 min intervals. The basal temperature is calculated by averaging the 3 measurements before treatment.

3. Inject different reagents into the marginal ear vein of the five rabbits respectively and record the time of injections.

(1) Rabbit A is injected intravenously with 5 mL/kg of pyrogen-free NS that has been previously heated in a water bath at 38 ℃ for 30 min.

(2) Rabbit B is injected intravenously with 5 mL/kg of endotoxin in NS pre-heated in a water bath at 38 ℃ for 30 min.

(3) Rabbit C is injected intravenously with 5 mL/kg of endotoxin in NS that has been pre-heated at up to 90 ℃ for 30 min, and then kept in a water bath at 38 ℃ for 30 min.

(4) Rabbit D is injected intravenously with 5 mL/kg of EP solution that has been pre-heated in a water bath at 38 ℃ for 30 min.

(5) Rabbit E is injected intravenously with 5 mL/kg of EP solution that has been previously heated at up to 90 ℃ for 30 min, and then kept in a water bath at 38 ℃ for 30 min.

4. Record the rectal temperature in 5 min intervals. After injections for 1h, then record in 10 min intervals for 30 min.

5. Calculate the thermal response index (TRI) and the fever peak (ΔT) respectively (see Appendix Ⅳ for calculation methods). Compare the febrile responses among the rabbits.

5   Cautions

1. The ambient temperature should be controlled at 22 ± 2 ℃.

2. Lubricate a thermistor probe with liquid paraffin or vaseline in order to avoid injuring the rectum and anus.

3. Insert a thermistor probe about 10 cm into the rectum and make a mark on it in order to keep the insertion depth at the same level.

4. Due to the time limitation, fever experiments are generally observed for only 90 min, so the biphasic fever induced by endotoxin as well as the whole process of endotoxin and EP fever wouldn't be observed.

6   Questions

1. What are the regular patterns in the endotoxin and EP fever (incubation period, heat type, duration)?

2. What are the differences in thermotolerance between endotoxin and EP?

3. What is the role of EP in the febrile mechanism?

APPENDIX Ⅳ: Calculating thermal response index (*TRI*) and fever peak (ΔT)

1. Method for calculating thermal response index: The vertical coordinates represents the changes in body temperature, 5 cm = 1.0 ℃. The abscissa represents the time, 1.0 cm = 10 min. The average temperature of the three measurements before injections is made as the intersection of two coordinates, and the abscissa shows the baseline temperature. Upward value is positive and downward value is negative. The temperature curve which is called fever curve in febrile response is made by plotting the temperatures from different measurements on lined graph paper. The area between the baseline temperature and the temperature curve represents the thermal response index which is termed fever index in febrile response. Thermal response index is a better parameter to represent the febrile response.

Vertical lines are made by connecting the points of measured temperatures for 90 min to the abscissa separately. The area between the fever curve and the baseline temperature can be divided into 9 trapezoids or triangles. Calculate their areas separately and get the sum of the total 9 trapezoids or triangles which represents the thermal response index (cm^2) for 1.5 successive hours and is shown with $TRI_{1.5}$.

2. Method for calculating fever peak: The value of fever peak is the difference between the maximal rise in body temperature and the baseline temperature. The fever peak is another parameter to represent the febrile response.

APPENDIX Ⅴ : EP preparation

1. Fix a healthy rabbit in supine position with a rabbit holder. The operation is performed under sterile and endotoxin-free conditions.

2. Expose the carotid artery surgically after local anesthesia. Inject 6 250 U (12 500 U/2 mL) of heparin sodium into the marginal ear vein of the rabbit.

(1) Drain blood into a 100 mL transfusion bottle with a No. 16 needle connected to the arterial catheter, then add two drops of heparin sodium to the blood with a No. 7 needle.

(2) Centrifuge the blood at 2 000 rpm for 20 min. Discard the supernatant (plasma) after measuring, then re-suspend the sediment cells in an equivalent volume of NS.

(3) Add NS solution containing 1 μg/mL of purified Escherichia coli endotoxin to the cells at dose of 2 mL/100 mL blood.

(4) The suspension is gently shaken in a thermostatic water bath at 38 ℃ for 18 h.

(5) Centrifuge the cells at 2 000 rpm for 20 min.

(6) The supernatant containing EP is collected in a 100 mL transfusion bottle and stored at 4 ℃ until use.

Experiment 4　Hypoxia

1　Objectives

1. Establish the animal model of hypotonic hypoxia and hemic hypoxia.

2. Observe the changes in respiration and blood color caused by different types of hypoxia.

2　Principles

2.1　Hypotonic hypoxia

The causes of hypotonic hypoxia are hypoventilation, low pressure of O_2 (PO_2) in inspired air and soon. The common characteristics are that the arterial blood PO_2 is below the normal range, as well as the oxygen content and the hemoglobin O_2 saturation fall down. During the experiment, the mice are placed in airtight bottles with soda lime (Fig. 2). Oxygen in the bottle is consumed by the mice while the carbon dioxide (CO_2) exhaled is absorbed by soda lime. Thus the PO_2 in the airtight bottle decreases gradually, while the concentration of CO_2 in the airtight bottle does not increase. This model is usually referred to as hypotonic hypoxia.

2.2　Hemic hypoxia

There are two main causes of hemic hypoxia: the decrease in concentration of hemoglobin (Hb) in the blood, or the decrease in oxygen-carrying capacity of Hb.

1. Carbon monoxide (CO) poisoning

CO generator is set up according to Fig. 2. A mouse is placed in a bottle linked to the CO generator. CO rapidly binds to hemoglobin to form carboxyhemoglobin (Hb-CO) that is unable to carry oxygen, and this leads to hemic hypoxia.

2. Sodium nitrite poisoning

The iron in hemoglobin is normally in ferrous state (Fe^{2+}). As a powerful oxidant, sodium nitrite oxidizes the iron in hemoglobin to ferric state (Fe^{3+}), forming a methemoglobin (MHb) that has lost the ability to carry oxygen.

$$Hb\text{-}Fe^{2+} \xrightarrow{\quad NaNO_2 \quad} Hb\text{-}Fe^{3+}$$

Via an intraperitoneal injection of sodium nitrite to the mouse in the experiment, the model of sodium nitrite poisoning is established. Methylene blue is a reductant (Fig. 5), which reduces the iron from ferric to ferrous state. When the mouse is injected with methylene blue immediately after sodium nitrite injection, the oxygen-carrying capacity of hemoglobin reverses to normal. In this way, we can disproof the oxidation of sodium nitrite and discuss the mechanism of sodium nitrite poisoning (Fig. 5).

$$Hb\text{-}Fe^{3+} \xrightarrow{\quad 美蓝 \quad} Hb\text{-}Fe^{2+}$$

3　Experimental materials

3.1　Animal

Mice.

3.2　Apparatus

Airtight bottle, CO generator (Fig. 6), graduated pipettes of 2 mL and 5 mL, forceps, syringe of 1 mL, scissor.

3.3　Reagents

Soda lime (NaOH · CaO), formic acid, sulfuric acid, 5% sodium nitrite,

1% methylene blue, normal saline.

4　Procedures

4.1　Hypotonic hypoxia

1. Place a mouse in a airtight bottle with soda lime (about 5 g). Observe its activity, color of the skin and mucous membrane, count and record the respiratory rate (frequency/10 s) and depth. Tighten the bottle and record survival time, measure the parameters as mentioned above in three-minute intervals until the mouse dies.

2. After the completion of all experiments, the mouse was left to open its abdominal cavity and compare the color of blood or liver.

4.2　Hemic hypoxia

1. Carbon monoxide poisoning hypoxia

(1) Set up the CO generator according to Fig. 6.

(2) Place a mouse in the airtight bottle, observe its activity, and record its respiratory rate.

(3) Pour 3 mL formic acid into the test tube of the CO generator. Then add 2 mL of sulfuric acid slowly so that carbon monoxide is generated. Connect the airtight bottle containing a mouse to the CO generator.

(4) Observe the parameters as mentioned in section 1 of 4.1.

2. Sodium nitrite poisoning hypoxia

(1) Select two mice and observe their activity, then treat the mice as follows: one is injected with 0.3 mL of 1% methylene blue immediately after intraperitoneal injection of 0.3 mL 5% sodium nitrite. The other is injected with 0.3 mL normal saline immediately after the injection of 0.3 mL 5% sodium nitrite.

（2）Observe the parameters as mentioned in section 1 of 4. 1.

4. 3   The differences in the color of blood or liver in different types of hypoxia

（1）Take a healthy mouse and put it to death with cervical dislocation.

（2）Open the abdominal cavity of the normal and the hypoxic mice, compare the differences in the color of blood or liver.

5   Cautions

1. Make sure the airtight bottle is airtight. Apply water to the interspace between the bottle and the rubber stopper, the glass tube and the rubber stopper if necessary.

2. Make the intraperitoneal injection accurately on the left side of abdomen to avoid the liver injury.

3. Connect the airtight bottle with CO generator immediately after the CO is produced to avoid the spread of CO. Do not seal up the tube exposed to atmosphere to avoid accidents.

6   Questions

1. What are the differences in blood color in different types of hypoxia? Why?

2. What are the differences in respiratory patterns associated with different types of hypoxia? Why?

3. What are the characteristics in blood gas change related to different type of hypoxia? What is the mechanism?

Experiment 5　Hemorrhagic Shock and Its Therapeutic Measures

1　Objectives

1. Establish the model of hemorrhagic shock in rabbit.
2. Investigate the pathogenesis of hemorrhagic shock.

2　Principles

There are three initial changes in shock development：①Reduction of circulatory blood volume. ②Decrease in myocardial contractility. ③Increase in vascularbed volume. Clinically, shock can be induced by many causes, among which hemorrhagic shock is the most common one. When blood loss reaches 20% of the total blood volume, the reduction of circulatory blood may cause shock. In this experiment, the method of draining blood is used to keep the blood pressure of experimental rabbit at about 50% of the normal level in order to induce hemorrhagic shock. After shock is produced, different therapeutic measures are applied to the rabbit, with the purpose of understanding the pathogenesis of shock.

3　Experimental materials

3.1　Animal

Rabbits.

3.2   Apparatus

Rabbit holder, BioLab-410 system, pressure transducer, respiratory sensor, a set of surgical instruments, bulldog clamp, artery catheter, three-way stopcock, plastic tube, 5 – 10 mL and 50 mL syringes.

3.3   Reagents

1% procaine, 3% pentobarbital sodium, heparin, 0. 1% heparinized saline, norepinephrine, anisodamine (654 – 2).

4   Procedures

1. Weigh a rabbit, inject 3% pentobarbital sodium at dose of 1 mL/kg intravenously for basal anesthesia. Fix the rabbit in supine position with a rabbit holder.

2. Clean the surgical field in the cervical region by removing the fur with scissors, and subcutaneously inject 1% procaine (3 – 5 mL) for local anesthesia.

3. Separate one side of the common carotid artery (Fig. 7). Ligate the distal end and thread the proximal end of the artery with a loose knot for later use. Separate the trachea, cut a " ⊥ " shape incision which is located 0. 5 – 1 cm below the cartilage of laryngeal protuberance (local anesthesia could be used as needed).

4. Separate the femoral artery of the lower extremity (Fig. 8). Ligate the distal end and thread the proximal end of the artery for later use.

5. Perform endotracheal intubation. Connect to BioLab-410 system through the Y-shape tracheal cannula for recording the respiratory frequency and amplitude.

6. Inject 1 mL per rabbit of heparin intravenously.

7. Insert the artery catheter with heparinized saline into the common carotid ar-

tery, connect the artery catheter to BioLab-410 system through a pressure transducer. Insert the artery catheter with heparinized saline into the femoral artery, connect it to 50 mL syringe for releasing blood.

8. Record the normal blood pressure and breathing waves as the baseline, observe the lip color and measure skin temperature of the rabbit.

9. After the stable blood pressure is obtained for 5 minutes, release blood from the femoral artery via the 50 mL syringe. When the blood pressure drops to 3/4 the baseline value, stop releasing blood and observe the compensatory responses of the rabbit (the changes of BP) for 10 min.

10. Continuously release blood from the femoral artery via the 50 mL syringe to 40% the baseline value and maintain this level for 30 minutes.

11. Inject 2 mL norepinephrine (75 μg/mL) through the femoral artery catheter, observe the changes of BP. When the BP drops back to the level before injection, give the second injection of 2 mL norepinephrine through the femoral artery catheter. The third injection of 2mL norepinephrine will be made when the BP drops back to the level before the second injection. Compare the BP responses of the 3 injections.

12. Inject 654 - 2 (10 mg per rabbit) through the femoral artery catheter, observe the changes of BP.

13. Make blood transfusion by inputting back all arterial blood released from the femoral artery and observe the changes of BP until stable BP is obtained.

14. Inject 654 - 2 (10 mg per rabbit) through the femoral artery catheter, observe and compared the changes of BP between the 2 injections of 654 - 2.

Observe and record blood pressure, breathing frequency, lip color and skin temperature of the rabbits in all the procedure of the experiment.

5　Cautions

1. During pentobarbital sodium anesthesia, inject the drug slowly. A fast injection may cause respiratory inhibition.

2. The artery catheter should be filled up with heparinized saline before use. 50 mL syringes must be washed with heparinized saline to prevent blood coagulation.

3. Feel the femoral artery pulse with your fingers to get the right position for the incision of the groin region and for the isolation of the femoral artery. The location of the femoral artery, femoral vein and femoral nerve are in a parallel arrangement and the femoral artery is usually located in the middle.

4. When inserting the artery catheter into the vessel, make sure that: ① The tip of mantle plastic tube is not broken. ② The sharp point of the artery catheter is as close to the distal end of the artery as possible. ③ Once the cannula enters the artery by 2 mm, the assistant must pull out the needle, and the operator immobilize the cannula at the same time to prevent mis-positioning. ④Continue inserting for another 1 cm, then carefully ligate the artery with surgical knots.

6　Questions

1. How to determine the onset of shock? What are the signs that can help with the diagnosis?

2. How do the three initial changes play a role in the development of shock? What are the correlation among the three initial changes?

3. What are the characteristics of the microcirculatory changes in the three phases during shock development? Discuss the pathogenesis and compensatory effects of the microcirculatory changes.

4. Use allergic shock and septic shock as examples, discuss and compare the possible mechanisms and therapeutic measures.

Experiment 6　Ischemia/Reperfusion Injury in Intestines

1　Objectives

1. Establish an animal model of ischemia/reperfusion injury in intestine.

2. Observe the pathological effects of ischemia/reperfusion in intestine on the systemic circulation.

3. Discuss the possible mechanism of ischemia/reperfusion injury in intestine.

2　Principles

Acute intestinal ischemia can be caused by clamping the superior mesenteric artery for a certain period of time, which destroys the structure of intestinal mucosal barrier and makes it lose the function of preventing intestinal toxic substances from entering the circulation. Then, let go of the superior mesenteric artery to restore blood flow perfusion and function. However, the damaged intestinal mucosal barrier results in more severe tissue damage due to oxygen free radicals and calcium overload generated by restored blood flow perfusion and oxygen supply, leading to more intestinal toxic substances entering the circulation, resulting in severe toxemia and decreased blood pressure.

3　Experimental materials

3.1　Animal

Rabbits.

3.2 Apparatus

Rabbit holder, surgical instruments, syringe, needle, arterial clamp, pressure sensor, BioLab-410 system.

3.3 Reagents

3% pentobarbital sodium, 1% procaine, heparin sodium, normal saline.

4 Procedures

1. Rabbits are given 1 mL per rabbit of 3% pentobarbital sodium intravenously at ear margin for basic anesthesia, and fixed on the rabbit holder in supine position.

2. Remove the fur in the middle abdominal wall to clean the surgical region. Use 1% procaine for local anesthesia in the middle of upper abdomen.

3. Make a 15 – 20 cm midline incision at 5 cm below the xiphoid. Follow the linea alba in the upper abdominal wall, open the abdominal cavity. Push the intestines to the left side to expose the right kidney and spine. With the right kidney as the marker, the superior mesenteric artery is searched along the spine and mesenteric root. The superior mesenteric artery is carefully separated and threaded for future use.

4. Remove the fur in the middle of the neck to clean the surgical region and one common carotid artery is separated under local anesthesia.

5. After heparin sodium is injected into the auricular vein (1 mL/rabbit), common carotid artery catheterization is performed, and normal arterial blood pressure is recorded.

6. After the arterial blood pressure becomes stable, clamp the superior mesenteric artery. Determine the clamping time according to the experimental needs. Cover the abdominal incision with a gauze. Observe the changes of arterial blood

pressure during superior mesenteric artery clamping.

7. Let go of the clamp after the specified clamping time to restore blood flow perfusion. Observe the changes of arterial blood pressure during intestinal reperfusion.

5 Cautions

1. Do not overuse pentobarbital sodium because it may affect blood pressure response.

2. Turn the intestines gently to avoid excessive pulling which may cause hypotension.

3. The clamping of the superior mesenteric artery must be firm.

4. After the release of the clamp, the blood flow perfusion may not be restored due to the adhesion of the artery wall at the clamping place, and the experimental target of reperfusion cannot be achieved. Use the finger to rub the clamping place to establish reperfusion.

6 Questions

1. What conclusion can be made from the results of the experiment?

2. Why can blood pressure keep stable during ischemia? But, why does reperfusion cause blood pressure to drop obviously?

3. Why does the extent of hypotension depend on how long the ischemia maintains?

Experiment 7   Acute Right Heart Failure

1   Objectives

1. Replicate the model of acute right heart failure caused by pulmonary arteriole embolism and excessive infusion in rabbit.

2. Observe the haemodynamic changes and blood gas analysis in acute right heart failure.

3. Discuss the possible mechanism of cardiac functional changes.

2   Principles

Systolic dysfunction of the heart and cardiac overload are the two main causes of heart failure. The latter is classified as preload overload and afterload overload. In this experiment, excessive infusion and pulmonary arteriole embolism will be used to increase the preload and afterload of the right heart. The change of cardiac function will be observed by determining the related parameters, by which the pathogenesis of heart failure is indicated. In addition, this experiment involves many pathophysiological processes such as hypoxia, edema and acid-base disorder. Through the observation and analysis of the experimental process and experimental data, the relationship between each pathophysiological process can be overviewed.

3 Experimental materials

3.1 Animal

Rabbits.

3.2 Apparatus

Rabbit holder, a set of surgical instruments, BioLab-410 system, blood gas analyzer, pressure transducer, respiratory sensor, carotid and femoral artery catheter, three-way stopcock, syringe, hypodermic needle, infusion device, central venous pressure monitoring device, stethoscope.

3.3 Reagents

1% procaine, 3% pentobarbital sodium, heparin sodium, heparinized saline, normal saline, liquid paraffin.

4 Procedures

1. Weigh a rabbit, inject 3% pentobarbital sodium at dose of 1 mL/kg intravenously by ear vein for basal anesthesia. Fix the rabbit in supine position with a rabbit holder.

2. Clean the surgical field on the cervical region and one side of the groin region by removing the fur with scissors. Subcutaneously inject 1% procaine (3 – 5 mL) for local anesthesia.

3. Separate one common carotid artery, bilateral jugular vein and one femoral artery. Trachea is then separated and intubated.

4. Inject 1 mL per rabbit of heparin sodium intravenously by ear vein.

5. Connect the respiratory sensor to the endotracheal intubation and BioLab-410 system to record the respiratory rate and amplitude.

6. Insert the artery catheter with heparinized saline into the carotid artery, connect the catheter to the BioLab-410 system via the pressure transducer.

7. Insert another artery catheter with heparinized saline into femoral artery and link a syringe by a three-way stopcock to collect blood for blood gas analysis.

8. Connect the left jugular vein tube to the infusion device and administer at a rate of 10 drops/min.

9. Determine the "0" position by adjusting the "0" mark of the central venous pressure monitoring device to the same altitude of the midaxillary line. Insert the catheter, which is connected to the central venous pressure monitoring device, into the right side of jugular vein. During the intubating process, the liquid level in the central venous pressure monitoring device drops continuously. When the tube is inserted for 5 – 6 cm, the liquid level stops dropping but fluctuates with the breathing waves. At this time, the height of the liquid level represents the central venous pressure. Then fix the catheter securely.

10. Observe the general condition of the animal, record a period of normal blood pressure and respiration curve. Auscultate the normal heart sounds and breath sounds. Measure the central venous pressure and blood gas values. Perform the liver – central venous pressure regurgitation test (slightly push and press the right costal arch for 3 seconds, record the increase in central venous pressure by cmH_2O).

11. Stab the marginal ear vein of the rabbit with a hypodermic needle. Use a 1 mL syringe to take liquid paraffin at a temperature of 38 ℃ and inject it slowly through the auricular vein at a rate of 0. 1 mL/min and closely observe the rabbit's condition. When arterial blood pressure decreases or central venous pressure increases obviously, stop injection. If these two parameters recover to the original level, repeatedly and slowly inject liquid paraffin until the arterial blood pressure decreases

by 10 – 20 mmHg or the central venous pressure increases obviously (The total volume of liquid paraffin is no more than 0. 5 mL/kg). Keep the auricular vein open with normal saline.

12. Repeat the step 10.

13. Inject normal saline at a rate of 80 drops/min intravenously 5 min later. Observe and record the parameters as mentioned above until the rabbit dies.

14. Push and press the thorax and observe the color and feature of the exudates from the trachea. Incise thorax and abdomen to observe whether there are hydrothorax and ascites; volume of the heart and cardiac chamber; external appearance and the cross section of the lungs; the volume of the liver and its external appearance.

15. Finally, incise vena cava to release blood and observe the changes of the heart and liver volume.

5　Cautions

The amount of liquid paraffin is the key to success. Over large volume or over fast injection will cause sudden death of the animal. However, if the amount or speed is too small or too slow, the effects of the injection will not be obvious. When infusion volume of normal saline is over 200 mL/kg and heart failure is still not produced, a small amount of liquid paraffin can be injected again.

6　Questions

1. What are the indicators of acute right heart failure in this experiment? Why?

2. How do pulmonary arteriole embolism and excessive infusion cause heart overload?

3. After dissecting the animal, what special pathological changes have you observed? How do these changes happen?

4. After the occurrence of heart failure, what compensatory reactions are possibly created by the body? Are these reactions present in this experiment? Please explain why they occur or why not.

5. What is the clinical meaning of central venous pressure in the diagnosis and treatment of heart failure?

6. This experiment involves many pathophysiological processes such as hypoxia, edema, acid-base disorder, etc. How do they occur? How are they interrelated to each other?

7. What happens to blood gas analysis when heart failure occurs? Try to analyze the illness by using the blood gas data.

Experiment 8   Respiratory Failure

1   Objectives

1. Establish the animal model of suffocation, pneumothorax and pulmonary edema.

2. Observe the different types of respiratory failure induced by pulmonary ventilation disorder, diffusion disorder and ventilation-perfusion mismatching.

2   Principles

Airway obstruction causes suffocation and induces obstructive ventilation disorder. The effect of pneumothorax on respiratory function mainly depends on the air volume in the thoracic cavity. Injection of small amount of air into the thoracic cavity causes slight pneumothorax with ventilation-perfusion mismatching. Severe pneumothorax results in severe restrictive ventilation disorder, with a significant reduction in total alveolar ventilation accompanying with ventilation-perfusion mismatching. The main mechanism of these respiratory failure models is hypoventilation. Diffusion disorder and ventilation-perfusion mismatching play a major role in the mechanism of respiratory failure caused by pulmonary edema.

3   Experimental materials

3.1   Animal

Rabbits.

3. 2　Apparatus

Rabbit holder, BioLab-410 system, a set of surgical instruments, Y-shape tracheal cannula, syringe, 50 mL syringe, No. 7 and No. 16 needles, three-way stopcock, spring clamp.

3. 3　Reagents

1% procaine, 3% pentobarbital sodium, 20% glucose solution.

4　Procedures

1. Inject 1 mL per rabbit of 3% pentobarbital sodium intravenously in the marginal ear vein of the rabbit to make a basal anesthesia. Fix the rabbit in supine position with a rabbit holder.

2. Clean the surgical field in the cervical region by removing the fur with scissors, and inject 1% procaine (3 – 5 mL) subcutaneously for local anesthesia. Make a cervical median incision and isolate the trachea. Cut a " ⊥ " shape opening on trachea where is located 0. 5 – 1 cm below the cartilage of laryngeal protuberance. Insert a Y-shape tracheal cannula toward the lung. Fix it firmly with a thread. Connect one branch of the Y-shape tracheal cannula to BioLab-410 system through the respiratory sensor. Record the respiratory frequency and depth.

3. Establish the model of suffocation.

(1) Clamp up the rubber tube connected to the Y-shape tracheal cannula with spring clamp to produce suffocation in the rabbit for 30 s. Record the breathing curves.

(2) Release the spring clamp, wait for 5 min to let the rabbit recover from suffocation until the breathing curves return to normal. Repeat the experiment 3 time.

4. Establish the model of pneumothorax.

(1) Insert a No. 16 needle connected to a 50 mL syringe via a three-way stop-cock into the thoracic cavity at the 4th and 5th intercostal space on the right side (a sense of sudden disappearance of resistance will be experienced when the needle gets properly into the thoracic cavity). Slowly inject 30 mL air every time into the thoracic cavity. Observe the changes in respiratory frequency and depth. If the changes are not obvious, continue to inject the air until the changes can be seen. Record the breathing curves.

(2) Drain off all the air from the thoracic cavity with a 50 mL syringe and remove the needle rapidly.

(3) Wait for 10 – 20 min until the rabbit respiration returns to normal.

5. Establish the model of pulmonary edema.

(1) Elevate the head side of the rabbit holder about 5 cm. Slowly (drop by drop) inject 20% glucose solution (2 mL each time) into the trachea through one branch of the Y-shape tracheal cannula. Observe the changes in respiratory frequency and depth. If the changes are not obvious, continue to inject the glucose solution as described above until respiratory changes occur. Record the respiratory curves.

(2) Clamp up the tracheal cannula after the obvious respiratory changes appear. Put the rabbit to death and open the thoracic cavity. Ligate the trachea at the crotch with a thread to prevent the outflow of pulmonary edema fluid. Cut the trachea above the ligation and isolate the heart and blood vessels carefully. Take out the lungs and suck the moisture off on the surface of the lungs with filter paper. Weigh the lungs and calculate lung coefficient.

$$\text{Lung coefficient} = \frac{\text{Lung weight (g)}}{\text{Body weight (kg)}}$$

(3) Open the lungs and observe whether bubble-like exudate effuses or not.

5   Cautions

1. All the air injected into the thoracic cavity must be drained after the pneumothorax experiment.

2. Do not inject glucose solution into the Y-shape tracheal cannula too fast in case of causing suffocation.

6   Questions

1. What changes of blood gas will happen in suffocation, pulmonary edema and pneumothorax?

2. What effects of suffocation, pulmonary edema or pneumothorax will have on the respiratory pattern? Why?

3. What will happen after repeating experiment procedures 1 and 2 for 2 to 3 times in the model of suffocation? Why?

Experiment 9　　Hepatic Encephalopathy

1　Objectives

1. Establish the animal model of ammonia intoxication.

2. Observe the toxic effects of ammonia and changes in animal's sensitivity to ammonia after most of the liver lobes are ligated, so as to verity the theory of ammonia intoxication hypothesis about "hepatic encephalopathy" and discuss the possible mechanism of ammonia intoxication.

2　Principles

The acute hepatic insufficiency resulting from ligation of most liver lobes combined with injection of ammonium chloride solution through duodenal intubation will result in the rapid increase in blood ammonia, thus the animal will show some symptoms similar to those of hepatic encephalopathy, such as spasm and coma. This demonstrates the pathogenesis of ammonia in hepatic encephalopathy. In addition, two control groups are set up. One is injected with normal saline instead of ammonium chloride solution after most of the liver lobes are ligated, in order to demonstrate that "acute hepatic insufficiency" is not enough to cause hepatic encephalopathy during the experiment. While the other, without ligation of most of the liver lobes, the animal is injected with the same amount of ammonium chloride solution through duodenal intubation, and will not show any symptoms. This demonstrates that the liver has detoxifying functions for ammonia.

3   Experimental materials

3.1   Animal

Rabbits.

3.2   Apparatus

Rabbit holder, a set of surgical instruments, syringe, needle, urinary catheter, cotton thread, suture needle.

3.3   Reagents

1% procaine, normal saline, compound ammonium chloride solution.

4   Procedures

1. Weigh a rabbit (hereinafter referred to as rabbit A) and fix it in supine position with a rabbit holder. Remove the fur on the middle upper abdominal wall, inject 1% procaine subcutaneously in the incision site to make a local anesthesia.

2. Below the xiphoid, make an 8 – 10 cm long midline incision in the upper
abdominal wall. Expose the peritoneal cavity and the liver. Press the liver downward, cut the falciform ligament between the liver and the diaphragm. Turn the
liver lobe upward, and remove the hepatogastric ligament by hand.

3. Use thick cotton thread to tie the roots of the left outer lobe, left middle
lobe, right middle lobe and quadrate lobe of the liver to block blood flow (Leave
the caudate lobe and the right outer lobe free).

4. Locate the duodenum, which lies along the pylorus of the stomach, and
make a purse-string suture. Make a small incision in the middle of the purse with

ophthalmic scissors, then insert a urinary catheter into the duodenum. Fix it with purse-string suture. Suture the incision in the abdominal wall. Fix the urinary catheter to the rabbit ear.

5. Observe the general conditions of the rabbit, such as the corneal reflex and the pain reaction.

6. Inject 3 mL of compound ammonium chloride solution via the urinary catheter every 5 min until convulsion. Observe any abnormal reaction of the rabbit and record the doses used.

7. Take a rabbit (hereinafter referred to as rabbit B) and repeat the above steps 1, 2, 4, 5 and 6 in sequence. This rabbit is used as the sham operation control group, except that the liver lobe is not ligated, all the operations are the same as rabbit A.

8. Take a rabbit (hereinafter referred to as rabbit C) and repeat the above steps 1, 2, 3, 4 and 5 successively. After that, 3 mL of normal saline is injected into the duodenum every 5 min to observe whether the rabbit has any abnormal changes.

5 Cautions

1. When cutting the falciform ligament of the liver, be careful to avoid injuring the diaphragm. When dissociating liver, try as gently as possible to avoid liver lobe rupture and hemorrhage.

2. The thread should be on the root of the liver lobes so as to avoid damaging the liver.

3. Purse-string suture should be carried out at the part of duodenal wall where blood vessels are sparsely distributed.

4. Prevent the compound ammonium chloride solution from leaking out of the duodenum into the peritoneal cavity.

5. Formula of compound ammonium chloride solution: 25 g of NH_4Cl and 15 g

of $NaHCO_3$ dissolve in 1 000 mL of 5% glucose solution.

6　Questions

1. What conclusion can be made from the result of the experiment?

2. Why can ammonia intoxication cause disorders in nervous system of the animals?

3. Can simple hepatic ligation cause hepatic encephalopathy? Why doesn't rabbit C show any symptoms during the experiment?

4. Why rabbit B with pure infusion of compound ammonium chloride solution didn't show any symptoms when the input amount of compound ammonium chloride solution is equal to the amount required for the onset of rabbit A? Will rabbit B develop any symptoms if the compound ammonium chloride solution is continued? Why?

Experiment 10　Acute Renal Failure

1　Objectives

1. Learn to replicate acute toxic renal failure model in rabbits.

2. Observe the changes in the contents of sodium and creatinine (Cr) in serum and urine of experimental animal, and to understand the functional and metabolic changes in acute renal failure.

2　Principles

Subcutaneous or intramuscular injection of mercury chloride ($HgCl_2$), as a nephrotoxin, may induce acute tubular necrosis and lead to acute renal failure.

3　Experimental materials

3.1　Animal

Rabbits.

3.2　Apparatus

1 mL and 5 mL syringes, 0.5 mL, 2 mL and 5 mL graduated pipettes, test tube, dropper, glass stick, table-top centrifuge, thermostatic water bath, type 721 photometer.

3.3　Reagents

3% potassium pyroantimonate, anhydrous ethanol, calcium hydroxide, 140 mmol/L sodium standard solution, 50 mmol/L picric acid, phosphate-sodium hydroxide buffer with pH 12.0, 2 mg% creatinine standard solution, 1% mercury chloride, 0.1% heparin normal saline.

4 Procedures

1. The rabbits are weighed and injected with 1% $HgCl_2$ (1.5 – 1.7 mL/kg) subcutaneously or intramuscularly 24 h before the experiment, then they are put in urine-collection cage and fed freely.

2. The rabbits' urine is collected for 24 h. In addition, 24 h after injection of $HgCl_2$, 3 – 5 mL blood is collected through a cardiac puncture, then serum is separated from the blood by centrifuging for 15 min at 2 000 rpm.

3. Measurement of sodium content by method of turbidimetry with potassium pyroantimonate.

(1) The pretreatment of urine: 5 mL urine is transferred into the test tube containing 0.2 g calcium hydroxide, and mixed with glass stick, then rested for 15 min and centrifuged for 5 min at 2 000 rpm. The supernatant, urine filtrate, is then transferred into another test tube finally.

(2) Measurement of sodium content is shown as Table 1.

Table 1　Measurement of sodium content

(unit: mL)

	Blank tube	Standard tube	Serum tube	Urine tube
Serum	–	–	0.2	–
Urine filtrate	–	–	–	0.2
Sodium standard solution	–	0.2	–	–
Distilled water	0.2	–	–	–
Anhydrous ethanol	1.8	1.8	1.8	1.8

(To be continued)

	Blank tube	Standard tube	Serum tube	Urine tube
Mix and centrifuge (2 000 rpm × 3 min), then the supernatant is transferred into another test tube				
Supernatant	0. 25	0. 25	0. 25	0. 25
3% potassium pyroantimonate	5. 0	5. 0	5. 0	5. 0

The supernatant is mixed and rested for 5 min, the optical density values of each tube are determined by a type 721 photometer (520 nm wavelength) with a blank tube set to zero.

(3) The calculation of sodium content:

$$\text{sodium content (mmol/L)} = \frac{\text{the optical density value of tested tube}}{\text{the optical density value of standard tube}} \times 140$$

4. Measurement of creatinine content by method of protein-precipitation with picric acid.

(1) The pretreatment of urine: urine filtrate is diluted at 1 : 50.

(2) Measurement of creatininecontent is shown as Table 2.

Table 2　Measurement of creatinine content

(unit: mL)

	Blank tube	Standard tube	Serum tube	Urine tube
Serum	–	–	0. 6	–
1 : 50 urine filtrate	–	–	–	0. 6
Sodium standard solution	–	0. 6	–	–
Distilled water	0. 6	–	–	–
50 mmol/L picric acid	2. 4	2. 4	2. 4	2. 4

(To be continued)

	Blank tube	Standard tube	Serum tube	Urine tube
Mix for 3 min and centrifuge (2 000 rpm × 10 min), then the supernatant is poured into another test tube				
Phosphate-sodium hydroxide buffer with pH 12.0	0.6	0.6	0.6	0.6

The diluted urine filtrate is fully mixed, placed in a 37 ℃ water bath for 25 min, then cooled and rested for 20 min. The optical density values of each tube are determined by a type 721 photometer (525 nm wavelength) with a blank tube set to zero.

(3) The calculation of creatinine content:

$$\text{creatinine content (mg/dL)} = \frac{\text{the optical density value of tested tube}}{\text{the optical density value of standard tube}} \times 2$$

5. The same methods as above are used for the determination of sodium and creatinine contents in serum and urine of the normal control rabbit.

5 Record of experimental results

Testing indexes	Normal control rabbit	Rabbit with acute renal failure
Urine sodium content		
Serum sodium content		
Urine creatinine content		
Serum creatinine content		

6 Questions

1. What are the nephrotoxins that cause acute renal failure?

2. What type of acute renal failure can be caused by mercury chloride?

3. What pathological damages of renal tissue structure can be caused by mercury chloride? What is the mechanism that leads to acute renal failure?

4. What are the characteristics of functional and metabolic changes of acute renal failure?

Chapter 4　Clinical Cases and Discussions

Discussion 1

CASE 1

A 16-year-old female patient was admitted to hospital because of diabetic ketosis. In the emergency room, the patient was in a coma with dermatochalasis, poor elasticity of skin, sunken eyes, tachypnea and the blood pressure of 90/60 mmHg.

LABORATORY TEST

It was revealed serum sodium of 151 mmol/L, serum potassium of 3.6 mmol/L, blood sugar concentration of 453 mg%, blood urea nitrogen of 36 mg%, blood pH of 7.2, $PaCO_2$ of 27 mmHg and SB of 16 mmol/L.

QUESTIONS

1. Was there any disorder of water and sodium metabolism in the patient? What category was it? Why?

2. Was there any disorder of potassium metabolism in the patient? What category was it? Why?

3. Was there any disorder of acid-base balance in the patient? What category

was it? Why?

4. How should the patient be treated? What should be paid special attention to during the treatment?

CASE 2

A 28-year-old male patient was admitted to the hospital with diarrhea and could not eat anything for three days. After taking medicine and rehydration in a local clinic, he did not show improvement.

The physical examination was remarkable for: lassitude, obvious sign of dehydration (sunken eyes, emptying veins of extremities, etc.) but with mild sense of thirsty, hyperpnoea, abdominal distension, muscular weakness of limbs and blood pressure of 80/60 mmHg.

LABORATORY TEST

It was showed serum sodium of 120 mmol/L, serum potassium of 3.0 mmol/L, blood pH of 7.32, SB of 18 mmol/L, BE of −5 mmol/L.

QUESTIONS

1. Was there any disorder of water and sodium metabolism in the patient? What category was it? Why?

2. Was there any disorder of potassium metabolism in the patient? What category was it? Why?

3. Was there any disorder of acid-base balance in the patient? What category was it? Why?

4. How should the patient be treated? What should be paid special attention to during the treatment?

CASE 3

A 56-year-old male patient was admitted to the hospital with developed pulmonary edema.

LABORATORY TEST

The blood gas analysis results: pH of 7. 22, HCO_3 of 20 mmol/L, $PaCO_2$ of 50 mmHg.

QUESTION

What kind of acid-base balance disorder did the patient have? Why?

Discussion 2

CASE 1

A 30-year-old male patient was admitted to the hospital because of fever, cough and general weakness. He was diagnosed as getting cold, treated by giving moroxydine, paracetamol and cough suppressant, but he didn't feel better and had a high fever above 39 ℃ for 10 days.

PHYSICAL EXAMINATION

It was demonstrated a body temperature of 40.2 ℃, heart rate (HR) of 90 beats/min, respiratory rate of 30 breaths/min and blood pressure of 126/86 mmHg. An enlarged spleen was palpable.

LABORATORY TEST

The results showed that the total white blood cell count was $3.5 \times 10^9/L$, and a blood culture for typhoid bacillus was positive.

The patient recovered after the treatments against typhoid bacillus by antibiotics.

CASE 2

An 8-year-old male patient was admitted to the hospital because of fever, nausea and dysphoria.

PHYSICAL EXAMINATION

It was demonstrated a body temperature of 39.3 ℃, heart rate of 122 beats/min, respiratory rate of 32 breaths/min and blood pressure of 90/60 mmHg.

Antibiotic therapy had no effects on the patient's condition. The child regularly appears chills and high fever every other day, and his body temperature is up to 40.5 ℃. After high fever, the whole-body sweats and the body temperature drops rapidly. Blood tests showed plasmodium vivax. He recovered after anti-malarial treatment.

CASE 3

A 15-year-old female patient was taken to emergency room because of a 36-day fever along with a 30-day swelling and pain in her systemic joints. During this period, she took antipyretic analgesics and antibiotics several times, and the swelling and pain of the joint could be relieved, but the fever still continued, basically not exceeding 39 ℃.

PHYSICAL EXAMINATION

It was demonstrated a body temperature of 38 ℃, heart rate of 120 beats/min, respiratory rate of 20 breaths/min and blood pressure of 110/76 mmHg.

LABORATORY TEST

The results showed antinuclear antibody (ANA) of 1 : 640, positive Smith acid nuclear protein (SM) antibody, decreased total complement and C_3.

The patient was diagnosed as SLE (systemic lupus erythematosus) and remission was achieved after hormone and symptomatic treatment.

QUESTIONS

1. Please make your diagnosis for these cases with fever.

2. What are the types, causes and mechanisms of fever in the patients above, respectively?

3. What are the mechanisms for the changes of body temperature in the three stages of fever? What are the features of heat metabolism for them?

4. What is the most possible cause of fever in infusion reactions?

5. According to the dual effects of fever on the host, what problems should be paid close attention to during antipyretic therapy?

CASE 4

A 14-year-old female patient was admitted by the outpatient as "fever of unknown origin". One day ago, she developed fever after swimming, accompanied by headache, muscle aches, loss of appetite, light cough without phlegm and vomiting stomach contents once, but no convulsions, abdominal pain and other discomfort.

PHYSICAL EXAMINATION

It was demonstrated body temperature of 39.7 ℃, heart rate of 112 beats/min, respiration rate of 28 breaths/min, blood pressure of 120/70 mmHg, be conscious, poor spirit, acute heat, no rash or hemorrhagic spots all over the body, pharyngeal congestion, bilateral tonsil enlarged, a few pus embolisms and bilateral cervical lymph node enlarged. Heart and lung tests showed no abnormalities. Abdominal tenderness, no touch of liver and spleen, no pathological reflex. Little urine with yellow color. The white blood cells (WBC) count was $14.7 \times 10^9/L$, neutrophils ratio and lymphocytes ratio were 81.6% and 11.7% respectively. After admission, antibiotics and infusion were given.

Chills, shivers and irritability occurred during infusion. The body temperature rose to 41 ℃, the heart rate was 128 beats/min and the breath was shallow. Infusion was stopped immediately, one intramuscular injection of promethazine was given, and ethanol bath was given with an ice bag placed on the head. The next day, body temperature gradually decreased, the patient was depressed and sweating more. Continued infusion and antibiotic treatment was given. After 3 days, the body temperature dropped to 37 ℃, and there was no discomfort except fatigue. She was discharged after 6 days in hospital.

QUESTIONS

1. What is the cause of fever on admission? What are the possible diagnoses?

2. What are the reactions of chills, shivers and elevation of body temperature during infusion? Why?

3. What is the significance of giving an ethanol bath and placing an ice bag on head?

Discussion 3

CASE

A 65-year-old female patient was admitted to hospital because of sudden precordial pain at night for 8 hours. She had a history of coronary heart disease and angina pectoris for 8 years without any history of hypertension.

PHYSICAL EXAMINATION

Blood pressure on admission was 150/90 mmHg, and acute anterior wall myocardial infarction was diagnosed by electrocardiogram. After thrombolytic therapy, precordial pain was relieved, but arrhythmias followed. The blood pressure was 70/50 mmHg. She was sweating, pale, sinus rhythm, and the heart rate was 126 beats/min.

QUESTIONS

1. The patient presented with reduced cardiac function, namely myocardial depression. Briefly describe its mechanism.

2. According to the diagnosis of coronary angiography, there was no reflow in part of the patient's myocardium. Briefly describe the possible mechanism.

3. Try to describe the mechanism of excessive production of oxygen free radicals during ischemia-reperfusion injury.

4. Describe how oxygen free radicals cause body damage.

5. What is the mechanism of intracellular calcium overload during ischemia-reperfusion injury?

6. Describe the principles of prevention and treatment in ischemia-reperfusion injury.

Discussion 4

CASE

A 27-year-old female patient, had a 40-week history of menolipsis, was admitted to hospital at midnight 1 a. m. because of amniorrhexis for 2 days followed by a 12-hour of paroxysmal abdominal pain, then a 2-hour of shivering.

The patient experienced morning sickness such as nausea and vomiting at the sixth week after menolipsis. The fetal movement started to be felt when she was in the 20th week of pregnancy. There was no colporrhagia in the duration of pregnancy. Regular prenatal examination had not been conducted. There was regular menstruation, no history of dysmenorrhea or amenorrhea.

PHYSICAL EXAMINATION

Upon examination, she was found to have a body temperature of 38. 2 ℃, respiratory rate of 21 breaths/min, blood pressure of 110/70 mmHg and heart rate of 86 beats/min. Heart sound was regular. The abdomen was distended and the fundus of uterus was palpable 3 cm below the xiphoid. There was severe tenderness all over the abdomen. Fetal heart sound could not be heard. Obstetric examination revealed that the vagina was unobstructed, but congestive. Amniotic fluid was in degree Ⅲ with foul odor. The uterine orifice was open to 7 cm.

LABORATORY TESTS

The blood routine showed that hemoglobin (Hb) concentration was 125g/L, red blood cell (RBC) count was $4. 2 \times 10^{12}$/L, WBC count was $14. 0 \times 10^9$/L with a differential ratio of 80% neutrophils and 20% lymphocytes.

TREATMENT PROCESS

After admission, the patient was treated with oxygen inhalation. Diazepam was given, 5% glucose solution with vitamin C and dexamethasone was also intravenously administered, which could relief shivering but had no effects on recovery of fetal heart sound. The patient still complained of abdominal pain. A dead fetus was delivered by artificial labor after uterine orifice was totally open. The skin of dead fetus was extensively sloughed with foul odor. The lost blood volume during and after the delivery was about 200 mL. The patient complained of unbearable abdominal pain and complexion became cyanochroia. However, the amount of the lost blood from the vagina was not too much. Fluoroscopy of chest and abdomen showed a great amount of gas was accumulated in intestinal canal but without air-fluid level. The blood pressure dropped to zero when she returned to the ward, with shortness of breath, increased facial blueness, hazy mind, no rise in blood pressure, HR of 140 beats/min, arrhythmia and no coagulation after abdominal puncture. It was suspected that the uterus was ruptured and hemorrhaged, and laparotomy was performed immediately. It was noticed that the uterus was intact but inertia. Mesentery had diffuse blood oozing. Gastrointestinal tract was severe swollen. About 3 000 mL of bloody gastric content was extracted by gastrointestinal decompression. 2 000 mL of fresh blood was transfused quickly and the uterus was excised. After the operation, the blood pressure fluctuated between 90 – 70/60 – 40 mmHg. Cyanosis was exacerbated continuously accompanied by diffusing plaque type bleeding over the skin. 3P test was positive. The patient was unconscious. Scattered moist rales were heard over the base of both lungs. After antibiotics, transfusion of fresh blood, fluid infusion and other rescue treatment, respiratory and heartbeat stopped at 13:00 on the same day, the patient was clinical death.

QUESTIONS

1. What diagnosis can be made based on the patient's history, laboratory tests

and clinical symptoms of labor? Give reasons and evidence to support your diagnosis.

2. What was the progression of the disease?

3. Why did the patient suffer from abdominal pain, shivering and fever?

4. Why was there an increase in WBC count as well as in neutrophils ratio?

5. Why did the patient's blood pressure decrease?

6. Why did the patient have diffuse mesenteric blood oozing and positive 3P test?

7. Why did the patient develop scattered moist rales over the base of both lungs and severe gastrointestinal swelling?

Discussion 5

CASE

The patient is a 27-year-old male farmer. Due to palpitation and shortness of breath after activity for more than 4 months, and edema of both lower limbs accompanied by fever for 2 weeks, he was hospitalized for 10 days after aggravation.

HISTORY OF PRESENT ILLNESS

14 years ago, the patient developed joint pain in his right knee joint, shoulder and left arm joint, without redness and swelling. Two years ago, he had a recurrence of pain in his right knee joint, accompanied by redness, swelling and systemic fever. In the past 4 months, he felt shortness of breath, frequent cough and sometimes bloody sputum after exercise. Left upper abdominal pain occurred suddenly three months ago and disappeared two days later. Half a month ago, the two lower limbs began to have ascending edema, palpitations and shortness of breath were aggravated. He complained of breathlessness and chest tight feeling when lying flat at night, which could be only relieved by sitting up.

PHYSICAL EXAMINATION

General examination demonstrated body temperature of 38 ℃, heart rate of 130 beats/min, respiratory rate of 25 breaths/min, blood pressure of 120/80 mmHg. He was well-developed, medium-nourished, good consciousness, cooperating with the examiner with a semi-sitting position. There were several needlepoint-sized hemorrhagic spots on the conjunctiva of the right upper eyelid. He had cyanosis, grade I enlargement of bilateral tonsils. Jugular vein was distended and the border of cardiac dullness was enlarged. A grade III systolic blow murmur and a diastolic rumble murmur were heard at the region of cardiac apex. The enhanced second heart sound was accentuated at the area of pulmonary arterial valve. Moist rales in both lungs were detected. Abdomen was massively distended. The liver edge was palpable 6 cm below the costal margin in the mid-clavicular line, and 7 cm below the xiphoid respectively with mild tenderness and medium-hardness. The spleen was palpable 3 cm below the costal margin. There were pitting edema on both lower limbs and clubbed fingers were present.

LABORATORY TESTS

Some heart failure cells were found in patient's sputum. The red blood cell count was $330 \times 10^4/mm^3$. The white blood cell count was $10\ 600/mm^3$ with a differential ratio of 81% neutrophils and 17% lymphocytes. Urinalysis showed 4 – 5 red blood cells per high-powered field and proteinuria (+). Central venous pressure was 19 cm H_2O and arm-lung circulation time was 12 seconds.

TREATMENT PROCESS

After admission, digitalis preparation and diuretics were given, and penicillin 800 000 units/day and streptomycin 1 g/ day were used to control infection. On the 16th day after admission, he developed pain in right waist. Three days later, dyspnea worsened and he was agitated. Scattered moist rales were heard over the entire extent of both lungs. Cedilanid and oxygen administration resulted in no improvement and the patient was declared clinical death at 10 p.m. in the same day.

AUTOPSY RESULT

The autopsy revealed as following: 1. Several hemorrhagic spots on conjunctiva of the eyelid; 2. Cyanosis of the lips; 3. Clubbed fingers/nails; 4. The cardiac volume enlarged; 5. Dilatation of heart and ventricular wall thickening; 6. Mitral valve became thick, short and hard, and adhere to each other at their roots;

7. The chordae tendineae became short, thick and hard; 8. The aortic valve became thick and short, and adhere to each other at their root; 9. Several grayish brown vegetations on the inner wall/surface of ventricles; 10. Pulmonary congestion; 11. Nutmeg liver; 12. Focal anemic infarction of spleen and right kidney.

QUESTIONS

1. What diagnosis can be made based on the history of present illness and autopsy result? Please give your reasons and evidence.

2. How did the disease develop? (including the causes and mechanism in details)

3. Why could systolic and diastolic murmurs at the region of cardiac apex be heard? How did they happen?

4. Why did the patient present with cough, shortness of breath and bloody sputum? Why could the moist rales in the lungs and the enhanced second heart sound at the area of pulmonary arterial valve be heard?

5. Why did the patient feel breathless and chest tight when lying? And why could the symptoms be relieved by sitting up?

6. Why did the patient's central venous pressure rise? Why was the arm-lung circulation time extended?

7. Why did the jugular veins distend? And why did hepatosplenomegaly happen?

8. Why was the patient's pitting edema in both lower limbs present? What is the mechanism?

9. Why did the patient suffer from the pains in left upper abdominal and the right waist? Why did the increase in white blood cell count with neutrophils of 81% and decrease in red blood cells count present? Why did urinalysis show erythrocyturia (++) and proteinuria (+)?

10. Why did the patient have a fever? What is the mechanism?

Discussion 6

CASE

A 56-year-old male patient with a 13-year history of recurrent cough and gasp followed by both lower limbs swelling for two years was hospitalized for his aggravated symptoms during the past three days.

HISTORY OF PRESENT ILLNESS

13 years ago, the patient suffered from cold, fever, cough with a small a-mount of white sputum at the beginning and then yellow sputum, which was improved after treatment, but recurred every winter and spring season or abrupt climate change. At that time, he was still engaged in labor work in farming, but the above symptoms aggravated year by year. During the past six years, he was suffering from palpitation and shortness of breath on exertion, which could be relieved at rest. During the past two years, the swelling appeared in his both lower limbs and his abdominal distended. During this period, he had mild cough and gasp with white sputum, but it became worse at night, mostly around 4 to 5 a.m. Three days ago, he was admitted to the hospital with cold and fever accompanied by yellowish sputum, cough and gasp worsening, poor appetite and oliguria.

PHYSICAL EXAMINATION

General examination demonstrated good consciousness, independent posture, mildly rapid respiration, mild cyanosis of lips and puffiness of face. Jugular veins were distended. Hepatojugular reflux sign was positive. Chest examination revealed increase in anterior-posterior diameter and widen intercostal spaces. Percussion showed a voiceless sound. The lung-liver border was at the sixth intercostal space.

Dry and moist rales were detected in both lungs. The apex beat was unremarkable. The border of cardiac dullness was not enlarged. Cardiac auscultation showed that the heart sounds were faint, no murmur was noted, but with the heart rate of 116 beats/min and premature beats were heard. The abdomen was soft but with severe tenderness in the right upper quadrant. The liver was palpable 2.5 cm below the right costal margin, while the spleen was not palpable. Shifting dullness test was positive. Pitting edema of the lower limbs was noted.

LABORATORY TESTS

The white blood cell count was 9 800/mm^3 with a differential ratio of 75% neutrophils and 25% lymphocytes. PaCO$_2$ was 50 mmHg, HCO$_3^-$ was 27.3 mmol/L, SB was 20.5 mmol/L and pH was 7.1. Liver functional tests were normal. Total serum protein was 3.7 g/dL with albumin of 2.4 g/dL, globulin of 1.3 g/dL.

The electrocardiogram showed high peaked P-wave, clockwise deviation, right ventricular hypertrophy, myocardial strain and multifocal premature beats.

The chest X-ray demonstrated the pulmonic artery segment was protruded, the right ventricular arch enlarged, the permeability of the lung field enhanced and textures of the hilar pulmonis became crassitude.

TREATMENT PROCESS

After admission, the patient was treated with antibiotic, expectorant, diuretic, cardiotonic and improved gradually.

QUESTIONS

1. What was the course of the disease?

2. How was the patient's respiratory status? What was the mechanism?

3. How was the patient's function of the heart? What was the mechanism?

4. What were the mechanisms for the development of breathlessness, cyanosis and edema in this patient?

Discussion 7

CASE

A 45-year-old male patient who was suffering from a 9-year history of chronic non-jaundice hepatitis followed by ascites and anasarca for 3 months. Diuretic and liver protectants were used, but he was admitted to hospital for sudden coma 1 day ago.

PHYSICAL EXAMINATION

General examination demonstrated the body temperature of 37.2 ℃, pulse rate of 62 beats/min, respiratory rate of 18 breaths/min, blood pressure of 80/60 mmHg. He was hazy and uncooperative in examination. Skin and sclera were mildly jaundiced. The palpations of the liver and spleen were dissatisfied. Shifting dullness test was positive. Pitting edema of the lower limbs was noted.

LABORATORY TESTS

Serum total bilirubin was 22.3 μmol/L with conjugated bilirubin of 8.2 μmol/L. Alanine aminotransferase (ALT) was 160 U, albumin was 3.3 g/dL, serum potassium was 1.96 mmol/L, serum sodium was 118 mmol/L, serum chlorine was 64 mmol/L. The feces were in black color and occult blood test was positive.

Ultrasound scanning showed the upper border of the liver at the sixth intercostal space. The liver edge was 4.5 cm below the xiphoid, and 1 cm below the right costal margin. The waveforms were comparatively dense microwaves or sparse tiny low waves, slight obtuse, and the ending waves were attenuation.

TREATMENT PROCESS

After admission, the patient was treated with arginine, sodium glutamate, L –

dopa, acetic acid retention enema, neomycin, correction of electrolyte disorder, diuretic, fresh blood transfusion, but without obvious effects. The patient was pronounced clinical death 1 week later. Some bloody efflux spilled from the mouth after his death.

QUESTIONS

1. What diagnosis should be made for the patient? What category did it belong to?

2. What were the correct diagnosis of causes and precipitating factors? Please give your reasons and evidence.

3. What kinds of toxins did take part in the pathophysiological process?

4. Why did the patient have ascites and anasarca?

5. What caused the decrease of serum potassium, serum sodium and serum chlorine? What did these have any influences on the central nervous system?

Discussion 8

CASE

A 19-year-old female student was admitted to the hospital on September 3, 1999.

CHIEF COMPLAINT

The patient complained of lassitude and somnolence for two months. In the past two weeks, she suffered from vomiting and oliguria, burning sensation of urination and facial puffiness.

HISTORY OF PRESENT ILLNESS

The patient developed frequent urination, urgency and burning sensation of urination 9 years ago for 6 months. After that, the symptoms disappeared, but her physical strength gradually decreased, and she could not participate in normal school activities. She developed "anemia" five years ago, and the routine therapies for treating anemia resulted in no improvement. Later the patient suffered from diuresis and morbid thirst. Three years ago, some "proteins" were found in the patient's urinary sample. She had a frequent nosebleed in the past two years. Over the past two years, she has become noticeably emaciated and felt increased fatigue. One year ago, she experienced an intermittent pain in the left lumber region for six hours, which could be partly relieved by lying on the right side. Then she vomited foodstuffs for three days, without fever, shivering, bloody urine and urinary calculi. She was hospitalized in November 1998 with a blood pressure of 140/80 mmHg.

The laboratory examination results were as follows: hematocrit was 23%, Hb was 7.5 mg%, blood urea nitrogen (BUN) was 117 mg%, plasma non-protein nitrogen (NPN) was 143 mg%, plasma creatinine was 7.6 mg%, serum calcium was 7.9 mg%, serum phosphorus was 8.5 mg% and SB was 20 mmol/L. The specific gravity of urine was fixed between 1.006 – 1.010. Creatinine clearance rate was 6.8 mL/min, phenolsulfonphthalein excretion test (PSP) was less than 2% for 15 mins. The result of X-ray exam showed general decalcification of the bones.

In the past six months, she suffered from shortness of breath after physical exercise and a rise of blood pressure with 160/110 mmHg. The X-ray of chest and electrocardiogram indicated the left ventricular hypertrophy. She was loss of appetite for nearly two months, accompanied by nausea, vomiting and persistent dull pain in the left pubic ramus. Since then, she suffered from mental fatigue and somnolence. In the past week, the symptoms above got worse due to "a cold", vomiting 3 – 4 times a day. The stool was dry and thin without pus or blood. The urinary output decreased despite normal water intake accompanied by burning sensation of urination and facial puffiness.

HISTORY OF PAST ILLNESS

The patient had a history of recurrent sore throat in preschool period. She experienced "a rheumatic fever" at the age of 7. At the same year, a tonsillectomy was conducted.

PHYSICAL EXAMINATION

The patient is extremely weak, pale, thin, listless, unresponsive but conscious. Mild facial edema, no bleeding spots in skin and mucous membrane were observed. Her body temperature was 37.2 ℃, blood pressure was 150/115 mmHg, pulse rate was 96 beats/min. The border of cardiac dullness was enlarged leftwards. A systolic blow murmur was heard at the region of cardiac apex. Lung examination did not find any abnormality. The abdomen was soft but with mild tenderness in the left lower quadrant. The liver and spleen were not palpable. There were percussion pains in both renal regions. No pitting edema of the lower limbs or pathological reflexes were observed.

LABORATORY TESTS

The results showed that the red blood cell count was $25 \times 10^5/mm^3$, Hb was 7.2 mg%, hematocrit was 21%, the WBC count was 9 200/mm^3 with a differential ratio of 85% neutrophils, serum sodium was 116 mmol/L, serum potassium was 4.9 mmol/L, serum chlorine was 77 mmol/L, serum phosphorus was 9.5 mg%, serum calcium was 8.2 mg%, SB was 16 mmol/L, plasma NPN was 268 mg%, plasma creatinine was 15.7 mg%. Renal function test revealed the specific gravity of urine was fixed between 1.008 – 1.010, PSP was 0 for 15min, urinary protein（＋＋＋＋）. There were quite a few pyocyte, WBC and casts in the urine. X-ray examination showed general decalcification of bones without pathological fracture.

After admission, although some active measures had been taken, the patient's condition continued to deteriorate. She had nosebleed for several times. On September 21, her blood pressure rose to 250/130 mmHg, plasma NPN was 284 mg%, SB decreased to 8 mmol/L. During the period, she had epileptiform convulsions for several times, gradually entering coma, and was finally pronounced clinical death on September 28.

AUTOPSY RESULTS

Autopsy revealed the following pathological changes: chronic pyelonephritis with acute attack, enlarged parathyroid glands, general decalcified and soft bones, the hypertrophic and dilated left ventricle of heart, mitral incompetence, colon ulcer and bronchopneumonia of lower lobe of right lung.

QUESTIONS

1. What is the clinical diagnosis of the patient? Please offer related evidence.

2. Describe the development of the disease briefly.

3. What clinical manifestations did the patient have? Why and how did they take place?

Afterword

The editor of this book is a highly qualified teacher with many years of classroom medical teaching experiences in theoretical and experimental knowledge. Due to the short preparation time, there are inevitably shortcomings and omissions. We hope colleagues and readers from the same profession can kindly provide us with advice and suggestions on revision so that we can further improve this book in the future.

The book has been reviewed and revised by Professor Daxiang Lu, Professor Yanping Chen, Professor Fang Wang and Mr. Keyao Bao. All these work would be impossible without the strong support and encouragement of the author's college and Jinan University Press. The authors also feel grateful to the students from International School and Medicine School of Jinan University, who unselfishly contributed their helpful discussions and opinions to the work.

The editor
March 2022